Praise for How Patients Think

"Dr LaFountain presents a provocative challenge to the business of healthcare and what we are aiming to achieve."

—Gabriel McGlynn,
Managing Director, Neubourg Pharma UK.

"A sophisticated handling of one of the industry's most pressing priorities."

—Charlotte Sibley,
President, Sibley Associates.

"A convincing approach to the progression of new models of healthcare management."

—John S. Ondik,
President, The Ondik Group.

"Congratulations to Dr LaFountain on raising the bar. We have been appropriately challenged to see things differently, and to do things differently. This will have a dramatic impact, not just on patients but on how healthcare executives go about their business."

—Sherrin Johnson,
Former Senior Director, Johnson & Johnson.

How Patients Think

A Science-Based Strategy for Patient Engagement and Population Health

Andrea LaFountain, PhD

Cover design by Zayrel Calderon on Facebook

For further information please contact
howpatientsthink@mind-field-solutions.com

The Library of Congress Control Number: 2016903996

ISBN-13: 978-0-692-66095-9 (paperback)

Printed in the United States of America

For all those who are called to a purpose of improving health; let our work be beneficial onto those we serve.

ACKNOWLEDGEMENTS

Special thanks to my advisors for their guidance
and support over the years, specifically;

Gabriel McGlynn,
Charlotte Sibley,
John Ondik, and
Betty Michelson.

Thanks also to those who have shared in this vision;
Sherrin Johnson,
Girish Patwardhan,
Sean and Marcie Catka,
James and Philomena Moran.

And most of all, my faithful family,
Andy LaFountain,
Matthew, Adam, James, Simon and Molly,
for their continued encouragement over the years.

Table of Contents

PART III

FOREWORD

Healthcare has seen many transformations over the decades from changes in population health, changes in treatments options and diagnostics, as well as changes in legislation and the administration of healthcare. Over the past three decades in my role as a practicing endocrinologist, I've seen a significant growth in the number of medicines and technologies available to treat disease. In my early career as an Endocrinologist, the treatment of diabetes followed a relatively simple process of diet and exercise, Metformin, and, if necessary, insulin. In recent years we have seen a proliferation of treatment options for diabetes with the addition of GLPs, SGLT2s, and DPP-4s. While these are all worthwhile developments, we have yet to make significant advancements in the control of diabetes at a national level. Over the past three decades, I've also witnessed a significant increase in the prevalence of diabetes and the volume of patients experiencing complications as a result of uncontrolled disease. Somewhere, in the progression of health, there is a disconnect.

Why, when so many great treatment options exist, are patients still living compromised lives due to sub-optimal health management? As providers of care, we have known for some time that not all patients embrace treatment decisions that are made in the physician's office, even when these decisions are the result of a two-way dialogue and, seemingly, mutual agreement between the physician and the patient. And while we know that not all patients embrace treatment decisions, we do not necessarily know which patients will, and which will not, manage their disease appropriately. This presents a significant challenge to the effective and efficient delivery of care and our ability to affect health outcomes.

Healthcare is moving in a new direction with an emphasis on personalized care and accountability for outcomes. We can expect to see even more attention on health outcomes as Accountable Care Organizations (ACOs) become more firmly established. In order to deliver against these new goals and significantly affect health outcomes, we need a more thorough and comprehensive approach to individualized patient care. We need personalized approaches that go beyond the conventional symptoms-diagnosis-treatment approach: we need strategies that operate from a deeper understanding of the patient.

Dr. LaFountain has examined patient decision-making from a cognitive neuropsychological perspective and shared some of her findings in her book. *How Patients Think* allows us to view the patient from the 'mind-side-out' using a scientifically valid approach. Her approach is not just for practicing physicians, but importantly, for business executives who are tasked with the strategy for improving outcomes at a population level. The strategic approach that is presented is evidence-based and thorough, from business objectives to return of investment. In a continually transforming industry, the next tier of transformation that is required is operating from a scientific basis of how patients think. Dr. LaFountain describes the pathway for that transformation.

Dr. Robert S. Zimmerman,
Vice-Chair, Endocrinology,
The Cleveland Clinic Foundation, Ohio.

INTRODUCTION

The cost of healthcare in the United States almost doubles each decade. It now stands at a tall $3 trillion per annum[1] with a per capita cost of $9,523,[2] up from $4,881 in 2000.[3] At this trajectory, in ten years the costs of care will rise to over $5 trillion. Currently, healthcare spend represents 17.5% of GDP,[4] consuming more than education (7.3%),[5] science and technology R&D (2.8%),[6] and infrastructure (2.3%)[7] combined. Is this an appropriate allocation of funding? Should healthcare spend be more than double the spend in education? Or over six times the spend in science and technology R&D? Spending on healthcare will remain a priority, but serious consideration of what is a justifiable and defensible spend needs to be given, and inefficiencies within the system need to be recognized and managed appropriately.

There are many areas within healthcare that require close examination. From the bench of basic research to the shelf of consumption, there exists a complex myriad of scientists, decision-makers, influencers, and buyers and sellers—perhaps more complex than any other market or industry. This book focuses on what has been recognized as the weakest link within this complex system and what has been singled out as the number-one barrier to achieving improved healthcare outcomes—the patient.[8,9] To be clear, this is not an accusatory attack on patients. On the contrary, the resounding message of this book is that patients need support: the right patients need the right support at the right time. While that's an old mantra, the reality of efforts over the past decade shows a serious failure to produce either improved health outcomes or cost savings. Current methods are clearly outdated, a fact that can't be ignored any longer. Patients are floundering under misconceptions of "health," what it means to be "healthy" or "sick," and what "good" health looks like for them, given their various conditions, socio-economic status, age and ethnicity. The healthcare system has simply failed to meet patients where they need to be met. This book is intended to shed light on where and why we have failed, and to provide strategic solutions grounded in the science of patient decision-making to advance new business models. As stakeholders in the design, delivery, and administration of healthcare, we have an obligation, from both an ethical and fiduciary standpoint, to empower patients to take ownership of—and be accountable for—their health. We cannot afford to continue with haphazard approaches to patient care and population management if we are serious about significantly changing the value and consumption of healthcare. It is our responsibility to develop and execute new evidence-based strategies of patient management that can effectively and efficiently deliver improved health within reasonable budgets.

This book implores all stakeholders in healthcare to leave behind the failed methods of the past and to explore, with anticipation and expectation, the potential of cognitive science as a foundation for patient and population management. It also presents a pathway to achieve this including how to formulate a scientific strategy for business, how to implement patient-centric solutions that simultaneously impact population health, and how to set business-relevant metrics with accountability for health outcomes.

PART I

THE NECESSITY OF SCIENCE
IN PATIENT ENGAGEMENT AND POPULATION HEALTH

Chapter 1: A System in Crisis—Straining and Loose at the Seams

In 2008, PricewaterhouseCoopers published a report stating that of the $2.2 trillion spent on healthcare in the USA, a staggering $1.2 trillion is wastage that could be eliminated.[10] They divided this healthcare waste into three major categories: behavioral, clinical, and operational. They defined these areas as follows: "Behavioral— where individual behaviors are shown to lead to health problems, and have potential opportunities for earlier, non-medical interventions; Clinical—where medical care itself is considered inappropriate, entailing overuse, misuse or under-use of particular interventions, missed opportunities for earlier interventions, and overt errors leading to quality problems for the patient, plus cost and rework, and; Operational—where administrative or other business processes appear to add costs without creating value." [11]

Across these categories of spend, the consequences of poor management within healthcare are far-reaching: insurers incur costs for managing disease complications that could have been avoided; employers suffer losses in work productivity and increased health insurance premiums; pharmaceutical manufacturers don't reach projected revenue targets, compromising the drug-development value proposition; physician practices fail to achieve health outcomes and lose out on reimbursement; and patients live compromised lives, further increasing the cost of care.

To deliver effective and efficient healthcare, a complex system of connected events is required. Pharmaceutical manufacturers need to develop drugs that offer a positive value proposition in terms of costs versus impact on outcomes; physicians need to make accurate diagnosis and treatment decisions; insurers/payers need to support reimbursement appropriately for proven treatments; patients need access to these treatments; and patients need to follow treatment regimens as recommended by their physicians. Inefficiencies can arise at any juncture in the system creating additional cost, loss of revenue and sub-optimal outcomes.

A WELL-OILED MACHINE—ALMOST!

Looking across this connected chain of events, at the earliest stage of the process, drug development, the United States is in pretty good shape. In some disease categories, such as lung cancer or

Alzheimer's disease for example, treatment options are limited, stalling healthcare improvement at the core until the discovery of new products expands treatment options. However, in most major categories of disease (diabetes, hypertension, hyperlipidemia, cardiovascular disease, respiratory disease etc), there is generally a diverse portfolio of products available to diagnose and treat disease and drive improved health outcomes. At the initial supply level then, the system is adequately covered.

Further along the chain, again we are well served in the United States, with highly trained and accessible healthcare professionals to diagnose and treat disease. In the United States, we have an average of 2.4 physicians per 1,000 capita, which is on par with the United Kingdom and Canada at 2.8 and 2.1 respectively.[12] Doctors are generally at liberty to recommend to patients a variety of treatment regimens that they believe are safe and efficacious choices to improve health. The majority of safe and effective medications and procedures are available to insured patients with modest fees (co-payments) and pharmacies are so widespread that 93% of consumers travel less than five miles to reach a local pharmacy.[13]

It would seem then that the healthcare system operates fairly well from drug development through diagnosis, treatment identification, and access to medications. This reflects the tremendous effort that goes into each step of this process. For example, for every 1,000 early stage drug discoveries made in the US, only one will result in the submission of an Investigational New Drug (IND) application to the Food and Drug Administration to pursue full clinical trial investigation.[14] The average drug takes twelve years to travel from fundamental research to the shelf[15] and costs a pharmaceutical company anywhere from \$2.6 billion[16] to upwards of \$5 billion.[17] Even with the appropriate financial backing, there are no guarantees that a successful clinical-trial pathway will lead to a marketable and profitable product. A major component of successful return on the investment in drug development is presenting a persuasive clinical argument to the FDA. The effort concentrated into this stage of analysis and documentation is astounding, with another couple of years passing between the completion of clinical trials and the FDA's final determination on viability. The FDA approval rate for drugs that do complete clinical trials varies from as low as 12% in respiratory disease to as high as 28% in anti-infectives.[18]

After FDA approval, making a drug or device available to patients at reasonable cost requires compelling contracting with insurers, in which every position on the formulary is hotly debated. Pharmaco-economic data is run through statistical models over and over to ensure that optimization of benefits is reflected in structured tiers of reimbursement and access; rebates are negotiated; volumes and/or outcomes are projected; and utilization is strictly controlled and monitored.

With a high-value product, FDA approval, and secured formulary status, the effort turns to on-boarding physician prescribers. This is another tremendous effort. Pharmaceutical companies must disseminate the knowledge through symposia that require strict peer evaluation of the clinical evidence behind their product, journal publications, marketing, and traditional sales-representative selling. The targeted physicians are carefully selected from statistical models of prescribing behavior, and sales representatives are trained and given lists of possible prescribers. Live data on prescribing activity across the nation is processed, modeled, analyzed, debated, and distributed. In the doctor's office, sales reps compete with each other for face time with physicians, getting their value messages teed up, and asking for the business ahead of the next guy who also will "detail" the physician. The calls get logged, reanalyzed, remodeled, reprocessed and redistributed.

Without a doubt, the effort involved in getting a healthcare product to the market is enormous. It is highly strategic and data-driven, and involves strong leadership, dedicated teams, and hard work. It's an impressive effort that is to be applauded. The race is being run with focus and stamina, the hurdles are being cleared with energy and determination, the baton shifts seamlessly from one transition point to another, the team is in sync, the finish line is in sight, the crowd is cheering, but then, at the final hurdle there's the fall!

The end result is a shocking failure to complete the race.

"Who put that there? . . . I didn't see it!"

"Sorry, I'm just the patient!"

CHAPTER 2: THE BUSINESS OF HEALTHCARE—WHERE IS THE MONEY?

THE VALUE OF HEALTHCARE

If it costs $5 billion to bring a new product to market,[19] in a market of 50 million patients, with 10% market share, and a goal of 3:1 ROI, then, to a pharmaceutical company, the value of a patient is $3,000 per annum. If "value" to a health plan is the average annual premium received from large employers for coverage, then the value is around $6,251 per patient.[20] If "value" is what the hospital collects for one inpatient day of care, then value of the patient is $1,791.[21] However we look at it, the value equation in healthcare is determined by patients' responses to, and within, the system. If patients decide to abandon treatment, there is limited return on the substantial investment in clinical trials, drug development,

27

distribution, and delivery, and elaborate actuarial models projecting the outcomes and costs of care become statistical trophies with little applied relevance.

COSTS OF MISMANAGED CARE

There are currently 29 million diabetic patients in the United States.[22] Of these, an estimated 48% do not follow treatment guidelines.[23] Within the Medicare population alone, over 5 million diabetics choose to ignore their doctors' orders and, instead, risk the consequences of uncontrolled diabetes, which include kidney failure, foot amputation, blindness, and cardiovascular disease.[24,25,26,27,28] The consequences of uncontrolled diabetes go well beyond the patient. The healthcare system is burdened to the breaking point by escalating costs. An estimated $245 billion was spent on managing diabetes in the US in 2012.[29] United Health Group published data estimating that the average annual cost per patient without type 2 diabetes was $4,400. With controlled diabetes the average annual cost per patient was $11,700, and in cases of diabetes with complications the average cost per patient increased to $20,700.[30] In a hypothetical health plan with one million members there are about 110,000 adults with type 2 diabetes. That's an annual cost to that one health insurer of over $1.6 billion – just for diabetes management! How can patient and population management strategy be applied to reel back some of this spend?

Getting to the heart of the matter, the patient, is not easy. Patients are the end users, but unlike in other scenarios, such as buying a car or a gallon of milk, in healthcare they are not the real decision-makers. They do not review their treatment options on a shelf, they cannot compare the relative value propositions across competing products in the market or review price points, and they are not the ultimate payer for the products they consume—in fact, they typically are blind to the true cost of their care. The seller (the pharmaceutical company sales representative) does not participate in any financial negotiations or make any contractual commitments. The decision-maker/physician (at least in terms of selecting the product from among the competitive set) often does not have any financial sensitivity to the pricing, nor does he/she consume the product he/she is selecting. The manufacturer cannot sell to the end-user, nor can the end-user buy from the manufacturer. The insurer is a huge middleman that organizes utilization across divergent populations that differ widely in how much they burden the system. Inevitably the patient gets lost.

PATIENT-CENTRIC FOR A REASON

Given the intricacies, effort, and expense involved in researching, developing, manufacturing, strategizing, designing, executing, and monitoring across the full spectrum of activities from drug discovery to marketing, one would naturally assume that a similar level of effort would be put towards that final critical component of achieving the end outcome—consumption by the patient. Dropping the baton at this final hurdle is unthinkable, but unfortunately that's exactly what is happening in healthcare today. The level of evaluation and precision at this final stage of consumer interaction is in stark contrast to what happens across the rest of the system and **this single omission is the leading factor in the escalating costs of healthcare and the low level of outcomes improvement across diseases.**[31]

Patient engagement has been suggested to offer *the* most dramatic potential for improving public health in the coming years; *more* than the development of new therapeutic entities and more than better trained physicians.[32] In the developed world, patient disengagement has become the new killer disease —not the lack of diagnostic devices, trained physicians or efficacious treatment options. Patients are actively choosing to discontinue treatment despite doctors' recommendations to the contrary. Even among patients with chronic conditions where mismanaged disease can have far-reaching consequences (e.g., cancer), a significant proportion of patients still choose to disengage from recommended treatment.[33] For example, a study of adherence to medication in patients with breast cancer reported that 26% of women with early stage disease terminated a 5-year treatment plan within the first year of treatment.[34] Other diseases report even higher rates of disengagement within the first year of treatment: Hypertension 28%,[35] Asthma 47%,[36] Diabetes 48%,[37] and Hyperlipidemia 55%.[38]

In investigating the costs of disengagement, one analysis suggested that Medicare beneficiaries with type 2 diabetes contributed over $3 billion per annum in unnecessary costs.[39] This $3 billion is wastage that would disappear if Medicare diabetes patients simply improved their adherence to medications by a mere 10%. That's a staggering return on a relatively small change in patient behavior. This equates to $120 billion in cost savings over ten years.[40] This estimate reflects only the *direct* savings related to managing diabetes. It does not include the additional savings achieved through reductions in cardiovascular events, retinopathies, amputations and renal disease that are associated with mismanaged diabetes. Factoring the growth in Medicare prevalence that will occur over the next decade, the actual cost will be significantly higher than this conservative estimate. The problem is not unique to the Medicare diabetes population. Patient disengagement creates similar unavoidable costs across all major diseases totaling an estimated $260 billion annually in the United States.[41] This vortex continues to gain force and risks spiraling out of control, if it hasn't already.

The costs (or losses) associated with disengagement are absorbed by inefficiencies across the whole healthcare system. Pharmaceutical companies lose out through patients terminating treatment prematurely and respond by channeling even more costs into marketing to steer more aggressively towards their forecast goals; pharmacies lose revenue and are more challenged to operate on a volume rather than outcomes business; physician practices lose patients (and reimbursement if they're under risk-share models); insurers who skimp on distributing care in early stages ultimately have to pay more later; employers have higher insurance premiums but a sicker workforce and reduced productivity; hospitals have to deal with inefficiencies and take huge financial hits from failing to deliver on Accountable Care Organizations' (ACOs) expectations; and patients are compromised in their health and daily living.

PERFUNCTORY MODELS OF CARE

Why are patients not compelled to actively manage their disease? And why have efforts to curb the problem consistently failed over the past decade? Why are co-pay programs, reminder tactics, side-effect management and wellness programs not effectively dealing with the epidemic of non-adherence such that significant improvement in outcomes *and* cost containment is evidenced at individual or population levels? Given the scientific and technological advances that have occurred over the past decade, surely we should expect greater improvement in health outcomes, *and* at a lower cost per patient. If it is true, as Dr. Kahn suggests in her editorial review of adherence rates in oncology, that patient engagement is the biggest contributor to improved healthcare over the next few years,[42] then arguably, all healthcare stakeholders stand to gain through improved patient engagement. The current infrastructure of the business and administration of healthcare has not delivered to this end. It is outdated and unsustainable. **A radical**

transformation of patient participation in healthcare must occur if significant improvement in health is to be a reality and healthcare costs are to be contained. This is not to be left to the patient alone; rather every stakeholder in the development, delivery, and measurement of healthcare is responsible for advancing improved models of care that are clearly and demonstrably linked to improvements in outcomes and cost containment.

CHAPTER 3: THE SCIENCE OF PATIENT MANAGEMENT

In his excellent book, *Predictably Irrational*, Duke University Psychology and Behavioral Economics Professor, Dan Ariely describes several entertaining experiments which illuminate the intricacies of human thought, decision-making and behavior.[43] One of the more interesting is his investigation into the way the *Economist* magazine structured its subscription options. He noticed that they offered 3 subscription options: "Online only" for $59; "Print only" for $125 and "Online plus print" for $125. It seemed odd to Ariely that two clearly different options ("Print only" and "Online plus print") were available for the same price ($125). Plausibly, no one would choose the "Print only" option for $125, given the obviously much better deal of both "Online plus print" for the same price. So why would the *Economist* structure its offerings this way?

35

A healthy curiosity spurred Ariely to run these scenarios by his students to assess how they would respond to these subscription offers. It turned out as expected. No one chose "Print only," and there was a heavy sway towards the combined "Online plus print" (84%) with a minority opting for "Online only" (16%). Where it gets interesting is when the options change. Given the obvious avoidance of "Print only," why would the econometrics gurus at the *Economist* magazine even bother including it as an option?

Ariely continued his experiment by re-presenting the subscription options, but this time he removed "Print only." Intuitively, and according to conventional economic theory, if we remove an option that nobody wants, it shouldn't impact the market. The results are shown below in Table 1. On this second presentation of the offer a dramatic reversal was observed with the majority now opting for the "Online only" (68%) and a minority opting for "Online plus print" (32%).

Table 1: Results of Experiment conducted by Dan Ariely on subscription choices

		% people choosing	
Offer	**Cost**	**Time 1**	**Time 2**
Online Only	$59	16%	68%
Print Only	$125	0%	N/A
Online + Print	$125	84%	32%

So why would removing an option that nobody wants have any impact on behavior, let alone reverse it? Several explanations are possible. Ariely explained this as the presence of the decoy, or the concept of relative comparisons across our choices. Whatever the underlying explanation may be, the experiment clearly illustrates two important concepts for engagement. First, decision-making is nuanced with underlying peculiarities, often subconscious and sometimes irrational; and second, if we can understand the nature of decision-making, we can direct the consumer decision to our preferred outcomes, as the *Economist* magazine did so elegantly.

THE SCIENCE OF HEALTH BEHAVIOR

Can similar concepts be applied to healthcare? Are healthcare decisions also nuanced with underlying motivators? If so, can these subconscious motivators be identified and harnessed predictably in a manner similar to that used by the *Economist* magazine? For example, can a patient's decision to disengage from his or her self-care be defined in terms such that we can intervene to direct the patient predictably towards the desired outcome of healthy behavior? If we understood the causal factors that explain differences between smokers who fail to quit and those who successfully quit, could we methodically steer the risk-of-failure group towards success?

In prior collaborative work with Harvard Medical School, the author analyzed engagement levels of women with breast cancer.[24] The analysis used data from over 10,000 women with early stage breast cancer. We found that 26% of women were not taking their therapy as prescribed after one year of treatment and this continued to increase annually to 38% at year two and 40% at year three. In the editorial comment regarding this study, Dr. Katherine Kahn from the University of California, Los Angeles concluded "*The empirical data presented...demonstrate that brilliant laboratory and clinical breakthroughs are only the beginning of the journey toward improved population health. To complete the translation...we need to understand the types of structure and processes of care that best support the initiation of evidence-based interventions.*"[44] Dr. Kahn goes so far as to suggest that "*adherence may be the most mutable predictor of patient outcomes,*"[45] raising the importance of patient engagement over-and-above the development of new molecular entities! Dr. Kahn suggested that if healthcare scientists saw their patients achieve the treatment benefits demonstrated in clinical trials, the health of the nation would be in a much different place. She asked why are we not seeing sharp declines in the incidence of cancer recurrence or myocardial infarctions given the plethora of great therapies that exist to treat cancer and cardiovascular disease? She concluded by challenging healthcare scientists to re-think their role in patient care.

Why, in a highly emotive and consequential disease such as breast cancer, would patients not be fully engaged in protecting themselves against a recurrence of cancer? Human behavior, and the decision-making behind it, is complex. Creating a change in behavior requires some acceptance of the evidence that describes the structure and processes that guide human decision-making. Advances in digital imaging over the years have provided opportunity to explore some of the intricacies of the brain-behavior relationship. At some levels, behavior is routine and automatic, while at other levels it requires forethought and planning. Different underlying cognitive systems underlie these different types of behavior. Routine behaviors (such as brushing teeth or getting dressed) are stable and remain relatively intact even under duress. The more complex tasks involving planning and decision-making are under the control of the "executive system."[46]

Researchers in the field of cognitive neuropsychology have identified several categories of behaviors that are at risk of suboptimal performance if not well managed by the executive system.[47] These behaviors involve (1) planning or decision-making; (2) error correction or trouble-shooting; (3) situations where responses are not well-learned or contain novel sequences of actions; (4) dangerous or technically difficult situations, and; (5) situations which require the overcoming of a strong habitual response or resisting temptation.[48,49] Health behaviors fall primarily into the first and second categories, and many fall into the fifth category (e.g. smoking cessation, dietary changes). Conventional marketing techniques work well for routine, automatic behaviors such as brushing teeth or getting dressed. However, with more complex behavior, such as smoking cessation or healthcare disengagement more broadly, marketing messaging alone will not have its desired impact. An intervention to change behavior will yield little impact unless the change effort directly impacts the system that is controlling the behavior. The status quo in patient engagement efforts falls woefully short of having any impact on the executive system controlling health behavior.

THE SCIENTIFIC METHOD APPLIED TO PATIENT ENGAGEMENT

Developing a program of behavior change in healthcare to advance patient outcomes requires at least three components:

1. Understanding the causes of patient disengagement;
2. Identification of those at risk of disengagement; and
3. Tailored solutions to moderate these "risk" cases.

All of these need to be pursued within the parameters of the scientific approach. Specifically, the field of cognitive science is at the core of human decision-making and provides valid and important experimentation on patient decision-making, motivation, cognition and consumer behavior. This evidence is powerfully leveraged in other industries as illustrated in the *Economist* magazine example earlier. In contrast, it is largely ignored in health behavior.

Why is such a rich body of scientific evidence not at the root of patient-engagement strategy and intervention? It holds many of the answers to our impasse in getting patients actively engaged in managing their own health, achieving improved health outcomes, and managing costs at a national level. And for certain, if we are to see a trickle-down (or up!) impact on population health, then it is imperative that the *sickest people* secure radically improved outcomes. This cannot be achieved with programs that operate at a surface level, programs that mask the real issues that lie beneath. We must get to the core of the behavior to create a radical impact that is detectable at a population level. For example, would the 84% of buyers in the *Economist* subscriptions illustration earlier have been able to explain why they chose the "Online plus print" option? Would they even have been aware that they were being heavily influenced by the presence of the decoy option? Perhaps they would suggest they assessed the value of each option independently, and that they are not influenced by such gimmicks as decoys. Perhaps they believe that they made an informed decision based on their own individual preferences of what represented the right value for them and nothing more. Recall that when the same options were presented alongside the decoy, the "objective" assessment of value was very different. It might not seem polite or politically correct to suggest that people are not fully aware of why they make the decisions they make, but the evidence is clear: awareness of our own internal brain-behavior mechanisms is extremely poor. In psychology, this is referred to as "meta-cognition"—knowing what we know. And because our awareness of these internal processes is a very poor proxy to the actual underlying mechanisms, we need to be very careful when we use a layperson's interpretation to understand how thinking occurs. This is especially true if the behavior is irrational or maladaptive (e.g., smoking, over-eating). Explaining our own behavior and the inner workings of the mind that propel us to do the things we do can be difficult. How then do we tap into those underlying motivators of behavior and harness them to create health? Thankfully, there is a wealth of science to help steer us in the right direction. The next chapter introduces how we can get the right patients into the right intervention at the right time via a scientific platform for patient management and population health.

If a scientific approach is not at the core of strategy, the years of investment and energy spent on population management will produce negligible return and little impact on health outcomes.

CHAPTER 4: HITTING THE MISSES—A CHALLENGE TO
THE STATUS QUO

Creating a behavior change obviously requires us to change
something. But what exactly should we change? The *Economist*
magazine example focused its effort on changing the consumer's
relative value proposition. It did this by adding a "decoy" offer that
would generate a relatively higher value proposition for the offer it
wanted people to choose. Chapter 3 briefly mentioned the difference
between behavioral psychology that focuses on our environment or
situations and how we respond to our surroundings, and cognitive
science that focuses on the internal mechanisms of decision-making,
which are the precursor to the behavior. Taking the latter
perspective of cognitive science, in order to change behavior we
must first identify the motivators behind the behavior and then
systematically change them. While this sounds intuitive, there is a
tendency in healthcare models of behavior to explain patient

behavior using irrelevant factors, such as demographic data (e.g. zip code, ethnicity, household income, and the like). This type of data forms the basis of most predictive models in healthcare today. Another common approach that is handicapping our ability to progress outcomes is a misrepresentation of segmentation models. The limitations of both these approaches are discussed from the perspective of behavior change—what they can and cannot do. A third barrier is also discussed, an over-reliance on patients explaining their behavior. This is a research dilemma often faced in psychological research where our subjects (patients, employees, humans in general) cannot sufficiently explain their behavior to a depth required for behavior change.

By holding strong to these barriers, we remain in the status quo and are prevented from progressing patient engagement and population health at affordable levels. Each of these barriers will be discussed:

1. Misapplication of claims-based models;
2. Misinterpretation of segmentation models, and;
3. Misunderstanding of patients.

After these three barriers are discussed, solutions are offered. Chapter 5 introduces an alternative, science-based approach and outlines a process for developing a scientific strategy for patient management. Chapter 6 details how this scientific approach shapes effective program design (the right interventions). Chapter 7 discusses how to apply this approach to identifying and profiling risk profiles (the right people in the right interventions). Chapter 8 outlines how to analyze the impact of this type of approach on the business of healthcare.

> **COURSE CORRECTION #1**
> THE PROBLEM IS NOT DISENGAGED PATIENTS,
> THE PROBLEM IS THE STATUS QUO—
> OUT-DATED MODELS FOR THE BUSINESS OF HEALTHCARE.

MISAPPLICATION OF CLAIMS-BASED MODELS

Claims-based predictive models are highly accurate when used to design and structure insurance contracts that are based on utilization in various populations. They can accurately project costs and risks, effectively determine appropriate premiums and pricing structures, and inform business negotiations and expectations between insurance companies and their customers. In this actuarial application, they excel. Unfortunately, they have been over-extended into patient decision-making and behavior. The problem is that these models are built using claims data that illustrate health activities (e.g., prescription usage) that are the *result* of the decision to buy/engage, not the *cause* behind the decision to buy/engage. This presents a real challenge to improving health outcomes, since even today's gold-standard predictive models don't explain why patients behave the way they do. Simply put, the data that drives poor outcomes (i.e., the data that explains patient disengagement) is missing from claims data. Consequently, models based on claims data cannot provide a basis for designing programs meant to change patient behavior. To the untrained eye, these predictive models appear to offer value, but their lack of association with the underlying principles of decision-making renders them irrelevant from a behavior change perspective. Furthermore, due to the fact that the precursors to the poor behavior are not evident in claims-based models, the identification of high-risk cases comes after the patient has already met some defined threshold of high cost, long after the window of opportunity for clinically relevant intervention has passed. This further reduces the potential impact on outcomes and diminishes the possible ROI from the intervention. The root-cause elements of behavior (or decision to disengage) must be the crux of patient engagement strategy. Claims-based models cannot do this.

> **COURSE CORRECTION #2**
> CLAIMS-BASED MODELS EXCEL IN ACTUARIAL APPLICATION, BUT WE NEED TO SHIFT AWAY FROM THEM AS A BASIS FOR BEHAVIOR CHANGE.

In sum, actuarial methods are misplaced as a strategy for behavior change and are outdated. They must be replaced by modern techniques that have an underlying basis in the science of patient decision-making and the power to effect positive behavior change.

MISREPRESENTATION OF SEGMENTATION MODELS

Models that describe segments are certainly valuable when appropriately applied. Marketing communication experts leverage insights on which consumers prefer digital communications, which prefer paper communications, and which prefer face-to-face communications to maximize the impact of their messaging. Clear preferences exist for verbal or visual presentation of messages, but the critical component when it comes to behavior change is not stylistic preference, but an understanding of the two or three key factors that cause the decision to engage or disengage. Segmentations do not explain why people in one segment differ from people in another segment. For example, in the popular "stages of change" model (also known as The Transtheoretical Model), patients are segmented based on their "readiness to change."[50] So the data is used to state that Person A is in the "pre-contemplative" segment and Person B is in the "contemplative" segment. The model does not state how Person A and Person B differ (other than by their group allocation). If we want to change behavior—for example change the behavior of Person B so he or she gets placed in a "better" segment—then we need to know the difference between Person A and Person B and use that understanding to guide Person B. Segmentations do not do this. The same is true of "personality health types." They are useful in determining the style of a message or *where* it should be placed (e.g., *Forbes* magazine or *Home & Garden*), but not in determining *what* the critical message should be. There is also a statistical reason why segmentation models should never be used for behavior change that is beyond the scope of this book. One statement only will be offered here to suggest the direction of that limitation: there is no dependent variable in a segmentation model, therefore the model can't identify the causes of the behavior.[ψ] We know for example, that young men in their twenties who drive red Ford Mustangs have more car accidents than old ladies in white Cadillacs. This is a segmentation of high-risk versus low-risk drivers. However, even though there are proportionately more red cars involved in accidents than white cars, it would not alter the true risk of the young, male driver to merely paint his red Ford Mustang white (i.e. changing the surrogate marker 'color'), or even to swap his car for a white Cadillac. In order to change his behavior, one would need to understand the factors that cause him to drive in a risky way. The true causal factors behind his behavior must be identified and used as the basis for change—changing the surrogate markers won't change the behavior. Describing behavior does not provide cause for action— explaining behavior does.

[ψ] For further discussion on this, please contact howpatientsthink@mind-field-solutions.com.

Over 80% of engagement solutions include a reminder plan that
costs millions of dollars to set-up and run. These plans are
considered a hallmark of adherence programs because, when asked,
patients state the reason they are non-adherent is because they forget
to take their medications. This is inconsistent with the data when
looking at pill consumption electronically (e.g., microchip
monitoring pill bottles). Forgetfulness is random, not systematic.
The data shows that the pattern of erratic drug usage that would be
expected if forgetfulness were an issue occurs in as few as 3%-8%
of cases. A more common pattern of medication taking shows usage
between Monday and Friday and then skipping weekends. This is
not forgetfulness. In fact, any regularity in the pattern of missed
doses is better defined as a deliberate omission by the patient—
something a reminder program will do little to improve. Describing
the behavior (pill taking Monday through Friday) is of little value
without the important explanation of why it occurs (e.g., the
patient's belief that "My life is my own at weekends").

Another common problem in progressing solutions for improved outcomes is an over-reliance on the patient's ideas of his/her thinking and rationale for his/her behavior. Amongst the thousands of consumers that the author has conducted research with over the past decade, the top two reasons cited for poor adherence are (i) side-effects, and (ii) costs. These also happen to be the top two reasons cited by physicians when they are asked why patients do not adhere to medication. However, objective data does not corroborate these subjective reports. For example, we see similar rates of non-adherence across drug categories which have widely varying costs, including generics; and highly toxic regimens such as chemotherapy have *better* adherence rates than more tolerable drugs such as the relatively benign statins. The top two reasons stated for non-adherence are therefore not the real reasons for non-adherence. Something else beneath the surface is at play.

Just as it would be inappropriate in the clinical setting of a physician's office to expect patients to explain why they are sick, it is equally so with behavior. To illustrate, suppose a patient goes to see her doctor. She has a pain in her belly. The doctor asks her to describe the pain and she can do so very well. She states the pain lies underneath her belly button, slightly to the left, perhaps she points to the area. She can describe it as a stabbing or throbbing pain, if it's worse in the morning or after eating. Her description is very informative. Now suppose the doctor asked her to explain why

50

she had the pain. Perhaps the patient would foster a guess, or perhaps she would stare curiously at the physician who should be making the diagnosis himself or herself. Of course the doctor would not expect to have his/her patient make the diagnosis; no matter how well patients can describe a pain or symptom, it is not within their expertise (typically) to explain it, or to self-diagnose. The physician understands that this is why the patient made the appointment to see him/her. The doctor, not the patient, is the expert at making diagnoses. After he/she makes a definitive diagnosis, he/she selects a treatment plan targeted to the patient's specific problem.

Now it should be the same with patient engagement. We can ask patients to describe their pattern of missed doses, or erratic exercise regimens, or how many cigarettes they've had in the past week, but we should not expect them to explain why they behave the way they do. Evidence shows that people can accurately describe their behavior, but they are, unfortunately, very poor at explaining their own behavior. In psychology, we refer to this research problem as the limitation of meta-cognition—we don't know what we don't know, or how our knowing occurs! Our over-reliance on patients' reporting of the reasons behind their behavior has led to millions of dollars being spent on programs that are doomed to fail from the outset. It is unreasonable to expect patients to diagnose the unseen mental processes that generate the irrational decisions that result in maladaptive behavior when experts in the field have been struggling to explain them for decades.

In order to change behavior, we need to focus on factors that we can actually change. Fortunately, the motivators that impact the decision-making behind the behavior are indeed factors that can be changed, so long as we can identify them. If we can identify and change them, we can steer the behavior in the right direction. The next chapter discusses how to leverage science to develop a structured mechanism of action (MOA) platform for designing targeted behavior change programs.

PART II

Charting a Course
to Improved Engagement and Outcomes

.

Introduction

In an industry steeped in science from research and development, protocol documentation, scientific symposia, diagnostics and treatment, it is not too far a stretch to imagine that same regard for scientific information flowing through to the ultimate end-user: the patient. This chapter presents a brief review of the scientific basis of behavior applied to patient engagement, specifically how patients make decisions around engaging—or not engaging—in healthy behavior. In order to develop and execute patient management strategy that is commercially profitable and translates into a measurable impact on health outcomes, it is necessary to leverage this field of science. Significant progress in patient engagement, population management and costs of care cannot happen without a change in our approach. Current methods have tapped out in their delivery of results. We need to go deeper, into the science of how patients think, in order to achieve positive results. Please don't gloss over this foundational step or write it off as "too academic" or "not my job." If your role involves the business of healthcare, then this is for you. The assumption here is that the reader has an appetite for disruptive innovation and a vested interest in developing patient engagement programs that challenge the status quo and deliver a positive impact on population health.

THE GOLDEN THREAD

Pursuing a scientific strategy for patient engagement and population health entails several steps. The golden thread that will run throughout the process is a strict understanding of what lies beneath the surface of patient decision-making. As a heads-up, this does not involve just using traditional market research and unfolding explanations of disengagement, or claims-based models. Instead, it entails delving into the scientific method, cognitive science and how the brain is hardwired to produce a series of decision-making steps, some of which lead to an engaged patient, and some of which lead to a disengaged patient. We will take a look at the basics of decision-making from this scientific vantage point and discuss case studies of how this approach has been applied in oncology, diabetes and ADHD. Some examples of application to smoking cessation are also provided, as well as a Science Selection Tool that maps scientific theories to particular disease areas (COPD, hospital readmissions, hypertension, etc). This shapes the who, what, where, when and how of patient engagement and its extension into population management. This approach also provides the continuous thread that links business objectives (e.g., to increase the number of patients >80% adherent or at HbA1c goal), with the process to achieve those objectives as well as the measurement of success.

STEP-BY-STEP APPROACH FOR BUILDING AND EXECUTING A SCIENCE-BASED APPROACH

Commercial strategy or health engagement efforts are only as strong as the foundation on which they are built. What follows is a step-by-step process on how to use science, particularly cognitive science and the mechanism of how patients think, to navigate us from concept to design, development, execution and measurement. The steps are presented in Figure 1.

Each of the four process milestones—(1) Develop the scientific platform, (2) Design the solution with a defined MOA, (3) Identify business relevant segments, (4) Measure progress to goals—is discussed in the next four chapters.

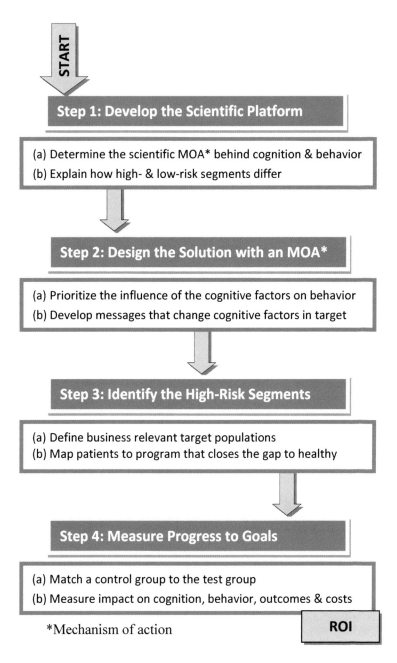

START

Step 1: Develop the Scientific Platform

(a) Determine the scientific MOA* behind cognition & behavior
(b) Explain how high- & low-risk segments differ

Step 2: Design the Solution with an MOA*

(a) Prioritize the influence of the cognitive factors on behavior
(b) Develop messages that change cognitive factors in target

Step 3: Identify the High-Risk Segments

(a) Define business relevant target populations
(b) Map patients to program that closes the gap to healthy

Step 4: Measure Progress to Goals

(a) Match a control group to the test group
(b) Measure impact on cognition, behavior, outcomes & costs

*Mechanism of action

ROI

Figure 1: Process for science-based patient strategy

CHAPTER 5: DEVELOPING THE SCIENTIFIC PLATFORM
—THE RIGHT FOUNDATION

Getting the right patients in the right interventions at the right time
involves finding the right patients, understanding their cognitive
profiles, designing interventions that operate on those profiles, and
matching the profiled patients to the appropriate interventions. All
of these activities have a common foundation—the scientific basis
of cognition and behavior. This chapter discusses how to construct
such a scientific model leveraging existing work in the fields of
cognitive science and health psychology.

Just as the diagnosis of biological disease allows for the selection of treatment options with specific mechanisms of action (MOA), so too behavior change treatments must be mapped to the pathway of thinking that directs the behavior. Fortunately, we have a rich body of scientific evidence available from which to develop valid approaches to health behavior change. For example, a quick search online for scholarly peer-reviewed articles on the psychology of health behavior returns a vast 175,000 articles! As an illustration, here are three that are relevant to adherence behavior:

1. Ciechanowski , P. et al. (2001). The Patient-Provider Relationship: Attachment Theory and Adherence to Treatment in Diabetes. *American Journal of Psychiatry*, *158*:29-35

2. Courneya, K. & McAuley, E. (1995). Cognitive mediators of the social influence-exercise adherence relationship: A test of the theory of planned behavior. *Journal of Behavioral Medicine, 18(5):*499-515

3. Avery, L. et al. (2012). Changing Physical Activity Behavior in Type 2 Diabetes: A Systematic Review and Meta-Analysis of Behavioral Interventions. *Diabetes Care, 35(12):*2681-2689

There is no lack of theories of behavior and cognition from which to design scientifically based patient management programs— programs that could propel our patient behavior efforts into modern-day scientific thinking and reel back some of the $3 trillion spent on healthcare.[51] According to health psychology, we develop mind maps, or schemata (sometimes called narratives) of concepts such as "sick," "healthy," "happy," "kind," etc. These are personalized and idiosyncratic, based upon experiences and expectations, with a flavor of societal trending in there too. If a component of health self-management is to take medicine when one is "sick," then it is important to understand what this concept of "sick" looks like. Anecdotally, some people consider themselves sick when they have a headache and can comfortably justify a sick day from work or a visit to the doctor. Others, like my father, don't seem to have a concept of "sick" at all. He worked a hard job in construction all his life, leaving school at the age of eleven to work and contribute to the finances of the family—perhaps he wasn't "allowed" to be sick, or perhaps he couldn't afford to be sick. I recall a time he came home from work, his hand gaping open to the bone from an accident with the saw. My mother was adamant that he go to the doctor for stitches. He bandaged it up with a rag and in his thick Irish brogue said, "Sure, it'll be grand." The next day he went to work as usual "without a bother." I don't recall him taking a sick day in his life.

The typical concept of "sick" when a parent is evaluating a child includes seeing overt symptoms such as fever, vomiting, diarrhea, or rash. An interesting question, for example, is in the case of ADHD. Does the parent of a child with ADHD consider his/her child "sick" even though the classic symptoms of being "sick" are not evident in the child? Could a parent justify pharmacological treatment for his/her child if their concept of "sick" does not apply to ADHD?

We were asked to develop a scientific model, or "cognitive architecture," of adherence to medication in ADHD for a pharmaceutical company. The hypothesis going into the research was simply stated: "Parents who treat their children with prescription medication for ADHD believe the symptoms of ADHD fall under a concept of "sick." And the converse of this: "Parents who do not believe that the symptoms of ADHD fall under the concept of "sick" do not treat their children with medication." Research was conducted on a large national sample of parents of children between the ages of six and twelve. Minimum quotas for "adherers" and "non-adherers" were set to ensure a broad spectrum of behaviors and cognitions could be measured. Parents were asked about their concepts of "sick" and "healthy." They were also asked about ADHD and whether the behavioral manifestations of ADHD fell under the concept of "sick" or "healthy." We asked about the role of medication and where medication usage fit within these concepts. Several other theories of behavior were also incorporated into the psychometric battery. A total of forty cognitive constructs were measured in over one thousand participants.

The results were remarkably clear and polarizing between the adherers and the non-adherers. Across the thousand patients in the research, 90% of the variance was explained. That is, practically all the barriers to healthcare decision-making were uncovered by the process. In other words, the specific differences between successful adherence and unsuccessful adherence were clearly defined. An extract of the final model is shown below in Figure 2.

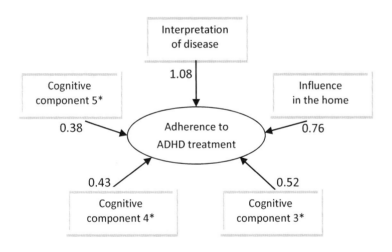

*For proprietary reasons, not all factors are labeled.

Figure 2: The Cognitive Architecture™ of treatment continuation in ADHD

Having a model that is specifying, *at a cognitive level*, the differences between adherers and non-adherers, opens up significant opportunity for behavior change interventions. I want to be very clear on this next point. Current models of health behavior change do not specify how and why engaged patients differ from disengaged patients. Instead, they quota (or segment) how many patients are in different buckets, without giving a scientific basis for the behavior in any of the segments. As such, they are limited in their ability to effect a behavior change (see chapter 7 for detailed discussion on limitations of Prochaska's Stages of Change Model).

In the mathematical cognitive model above, parents who understood that ADHD has a biochemical basis maintained adherence over a longer term. In contrast, those who believed that ADHD was a "behavioral" problem did not adhere to pharmacological treatment. Having developed this understanding and depicted the pathway of the decision (just as we would depict the pathway of a disease), we now have the ability to create a diagnostic tool to identify the cases that evidence the "disengaged" pathway of decision-making. For example, one of the strongest items on the diagnostic tool tapped into the dimension of "misinterpretation of disease etiology" with a simple statement: "I believe I can manage my child's behavior through discipline alone." To respond, parents selected a number on a 5-point Likert-type scale that ranged from "strongly agree" to "strongly disagree." If a parent agreed with, or was neutral towards, the statement, he/she was at high-risk for discontinuing the child's treatment for ADHD within the first 90 days of therapy.

Another important aspect of a scientific platform is that the *solution* to change the behavior is clearly marked out—just as prescription treatments for diseases have a mechanism of action that is clearly aligned within the pathway of disease. The communication that the parent needs in this ADHD example in order to bring about adherent behavior is a compelling portrayal of the underlying biochemical nature of ADHD. Failure to persuade the parent on this single dimension means she is unlikely to continue prescription medication for her child.

In the field of healthcare, it is important to maintain the centrality of science around the total patient experience—from diagnosis to the end consumption of treatment and the attainment of improved health outcomes. Cognitive science allows us to do this. The parallels between a biomedical model of the treatment of disease, with which we are all familiar, and a cognitive model of the treatment of behavior are illustrated in Table 2.

Table 2: Parallel between Biomedical model of Disease and Cognitive model of Behavior

Presentation	Marker	Diagnostic	MOA	Treatment	Follow-up
Diabetes (biomedical)	HbA1c > 7% mmol/moL	Blood assay	Insufficient glucose metabolism	Boost glucose metabolism (e.g.DPP-4)	Re-run biomarker diagnostic to check for change
Disengaged (cognitive)	Abandoned Rx	Cognitive profile	Misinterpretation of disease etiology	Education on correct nature of disease	Re-run cognitive diagnostic to check for change

So how do we determine the mechanism of action behind a behavior? Table 3 provides a Science Selection Tool (SST) to help identify which theoretical models are considered relevant for different health behavior applications. These models can be applied to many areas of health decision-making, including adherence to long-term medications, post-surgical care, COPD, weight loss, smoking cessation, vaccinations, etc. This list is not comprehensive—as mentioned earlier, there are many scientific explanations of behavior—but it presents some of the major theories that have stood the test of time, are easily interpretable, and have very strong application to health behavior. Different theories can work synergistically, and even be additive, further enhancing the power of any individual model, and increasing the likelihood of success in behavior change.

ONE SIZE DOES NOT FIT ALL

A question that is often asked is "Are the factors impacting adherence, or healthcare decision-making, the same for different diseases?" Unfortunately, they are not. It is entirely plausible for a patient to have radically different engagement profiles across different diseases. For example, a patient with breast cancer who also has diabetes may be very motivated to treat cancer with surgery, radiation, chemotherapy and oral medication to reduce the risk of recurrence. This same patient may have a very different perspective of diabetes, believing that the risk of complications (such as amputation or blindness) are not as real, and therefore may

Table 3: Science Selection Tool (SST) for science-based intervention design

Condition	Scientific Approach	Basic Tenets
Smoking cessation	Health Belief Model (Rosenstock, 1974)	Health behavior is predicated on the balance of value of the benefits of the risky behavior compared to the benefits of the healthy behavior. Also the risks of the risky behavior and healthy behavior are compared.
Post-surgical care (30-day readmissions)	Theory of Planned Behavior (Ajzen, 1985)	Behavior is predicted by the attitude towards the behavior (e.g., wound cleaning), the belief in one's ability to effectively conduct the activity, and the expectations that others have of oneself (i.e., to look after oneself after hospitalization).
Respiratory disease	Expected Value Theory (Palmgreen, 1984)	Behavior is the result of the lower projected probability of the high intensity outcome (e.g., exacerbation) versus the higher probability of the lower intensity outcome (normal day-to-day functioning).
Diabetes	Protection Motivation Theory (Rogers, 1983)	Behavior is predicated upon the perceived severity of poor disease outcomes and the belief that healthy behavior can effectively mitigate the poor outcome.
ADHD	Mental Representation of Health (Leventhal, Meyer, Nerenz, 1980)	Health behavior is determined by the concept of "healthy." Diseases that have no overt manifestation (fever, rash, vomiting) are not interpreted as having a biological basis, and thus require behavioral, rather than pharmacological, intervention.
Oncology	Locus of Control (Rotter, 1990)	Health engagement is determined by a belief that a strong commitment to change will create the desired outcome.

Copyright © 2016 Mind Field Solutions Corp.

not be so motivated to treat the disease. The converse is also true. For example, we have seen in our research that a patient with breast cancer can perceive that he/she has little control over whether the cancer recurs and, as such, not be fully motivated to treat it. Meanwhile this same patient could interpret the threat of diabetes to be more real and treat it aggressively by daily monitoring his/her blood and aim for controlled HbA1c.

There are, of course, a few exceptions to this. Those conditions that directly impact the cognitive system itself have wide, systematic impact (e.g., Alzheimer's disease, schizophrenia, depression, anxicty). These diseases can be expected to impact health behavior across all conditions the patient experiences. For example, depression has a globally apathetic impact on the cognitive system. Patients with depression lack motivation across most facets of their lives—sexual behavior, nutrition, exercise, occupation, social engagements, and yes—healthcare engagement. This is not the case with conditions that are neutral in their impact on the cognitive system (e.g., diabetes, hypertension, asthma, post-surgical cardiac care). Generally speaking, it is safe to assume that patients who have a variety of different conditions are likely to have a variety of behavior patterns across their conditions.

The reason for the variation is because the mechanism of action for behavior (or engagement) is different across diseases. For example, in ADHD, the interpretation of whether the condition is biochemical versus behavioral is a key factor. This is not the case in oncology, where awareness of the biochemical nature of cancer is very high. Also in oncology, the experience of having a family member with cancer heightens a patient's adherence to medication. In diabetes, the opposite is true. Having a family member with diabetes, and seeing a poor regimen of diet, exercise and treatment in that family member without complications, fosters a false sense of security that complications are not going to occur in the patient either.

The learning here is that we cannot make assumptions on transferability of models from one disease to another. Very different mechanisms of action are at play and it is important to uncover these mechanisms for each disease in order to have a defined, predictable, and successful impact in redirecting the course of behavior.

SCIENTIFIC RESOURCE ALLOCATION

From a resource allocation perspective, the following is an important note. The scientific method states that hypotheses must be stated *a priori*, that is, before the research begins. It also states that the intent of the surveying or measurement is to try to *falsify* research assumptions rather than seek confirmatory data. The reason this is important is that if faulty thinking isn't challenged sufficiently, it becomes mainstream "wisdom," whereupon it qualifies for millions of dollars of investment around program development and marketing. If the purpose of the insight is to provide a secure foundation for significant spending in program design and execution that will create a positive impact on behavior and a positive financial ROI, then purging faulty assumptions *ahead* of the spend is critical to success and the generation of a positive return on investment. In essence, data can confirm good and bad ideas equally. Bad ideas will come home to roost at some point. Purging them *before* they consume resources is appropriate. In the case example of this ADHD research, we were charged with developing a mathematical model of how parents think about ADHD and its treatment. Every false assumption entering the mathematical model weakened the overall ability of the model to function, and our ability to deliver results. We could not carry that risk into analysis—and the client couldn't carry that risk into faulty program design, spending millions of dollars that couldn't deliver results.

~   ~   ~

In summary, defining the mechanism of action of behavior—or more correctly, **the decision to disengage**—involves taking valid *theoretical* approaches to *cognition* and behavior, constructing testable *hypotheses* prior to investigation, and *testing,* via efforts, to falsify the hypotheses. This can yield a scientific framework from which to (a) construct a predictive model; (b) develop a diagnostic tool to isolate at-risk profiles, and; (c) provide training for patient support teams on translating these components of cognition into communication pieces for behavior change. The results are improved engagement, healthier outcomes and a significant improvement in program ROI.

THE IMPORTANCE OF DIFFERENTIATION

Before moving into the design of behavior change programs, it is critically important that program developers have a clear line of sight to the points of differentiation between the good (e.g., engaged, controlled disease) and the bad (e.g., disengaged, uncontrolled disease). The fundamental goal of every behavior change program should be to close the gap between the "good" segments and the "bad" segments (obviously by improving the performance in the "bad" segments towards that in the "good" ones). [Ψ] This requires a knowledge base of how the "good" and "bad" segments are different. It is this knowledge base that becomes the pivot for the behavior change, and hopefully, it is derived from a concerted effort that leverages the theory of behavior described above.

What we see happening in healthcare is actually contrary to this. For example, the vast majority, around 98%, of patients report that prescription medication costs too much. Even though many patients are on co-pay reduction programs and are paying a fraction of the

---

[Ψ] Chapter 7 presents a critique of current approaches that select "healthier" segments as the targets for behavior support programs. This is counter to the philosophy of behavior change and a primary reason for the continued lack of impact at a population level.

cost, patients still report price sensitivity. Specifically, when asked why they stopped taking medication, "cost" is right up there along with side effects as a reason for discontinuation. Typically in market research, if such a majority swing were found in the data, the report would contain a large print headline "98% of patients state cost is a barrier to adherence." The seemingly intuitive response to this would be to offer some type of cost-cutting program, for example co-pay support or coupons.

However, from a behavior change perspective, this runs contrary to what we are aiming to achieve. If all patients say cost is a barrier, then it cannot be a predictor of poor behavior. While this clearly goes against the status quo of how traditional market research is used for decision-making in commercial strategy, when it comes to behavior change, **only factors that *differentiate* engaged from disengaged can be used as a basis for *change*.** That is, if everyone (the engaged and the disengaged alike) reports the same issue (e.g., cost) as a barrier, then by definition, this is not a differentiator when it comes to the different behaviors we observe. This is true of any factor where everyone scores the same. From a predictive modeling perspective, it would return a near zero coefficient.

We can therefore, expect cost to have a very modest impact on adherence, confined only to the 5% to 8% of patients who have a genuine financial need. The return on investment (ROI) from cost/co-pay reduction initiatives bears this out. The ROI from cost/co-pay programs would be greatly enhanced if these programs were reserved for the 5% to 8% of low socio-economic-status (SES) groups that truly need financial support. Issuing them more broadly in response to the general consumer response of high-cost drugs, will yield little-to-no return and only serve to dilute the efficiency of the effort where it is having an impact.

So rather than cost being a true motivator for behavior (and thus behavior change), if all respondents agree that it is a barrier, then it could be managed as a friendly consumer-relations tactic to offer co-pay support, but doing so will have zero impact on adherence behavior because cost is *not* a factor that causes the difference in the behavior of the engaged and the disengaged. Yes, this is counter to the conventional wisdom of marketing. However, if behavior change is the ultimate goal, efforts *must* be focused only on those factors that clearly *differentiate* the desired behavior from the undesired behavior. Cost simply does not do this, therefore, it cannot be an agent of change.

COURSE CORRECTION #5:
IF EVERYONE AGREES, THEN IT'S A RED HERRING.
WE MUST OPERATE ON THE *DIFFERENCES*
IN ORDER TO CLOSE THE GAP.

The next section discusses how to prioritize various factors within a model—those that are causing the difference in behavior. We will learn how to extract the most meaningful factors for behavior change and thus maximize the impact of programs and secure a strong ROI from patient support initiatives.

CHAPTER 6: DESIGNING SOLUTIONS WITH A DEFINED
MOA—THE RIGHT INTERVENTION

When we look at examples such as the *Economist* magazine
subscriptions presented earlier, it is evident that consumer
motivation is not always logical. But it is understandable and
malleable. The example illustrated how consumer behavior could be
reversed through a simple change in how the offer was presented.
Interestingly, the offer itself, and the price points did not actually
change across the two scenarios, but nonetheless, the behavior
changed dramatically. The *Economist* business gurus could effect
this behavior change because they understood the essence of the
financial trade-off the consumers were making and they harnessed
this to meet their business objectives.

In order to create a change in behavior, we must understand enough
of the behavior to tip the balance and create a meaningful impact. In
the ADHD case study mentioned in the previous chapter, a
cognitive model was developed that resulted in 90% of the variance
in behavior being explained. That's certainly enough to tip the
balance—assuming decent execution of tactics. By understanding
the different cognitive profiles of the parents of six-to-twelve-year-
old children with ADHD, we were able to accurately state who had
a non-adherent profile, and why they were at risk of discontinuing
treatment of the child with prescription medication.

In contrast, consider the typical explanatory power of predictive
models used in healthcare today. A typical model might explain
only as much as 23% of the variance in behavior. This means 77%
of behavior is left unaccounted for, and thus is outside the remit of
influence of a behavior change program. A model that explains 23%
of the variance is insufficient to tip the balance in unhealthy
behavior and create a positive change. Even with perfect execution
of a premium patient support program, if 77% of the variance that
causes the behavior is left untapped, then the patients are unlikely to
change.

One reason the power of current models is so low is that the models don't leverage the true insights into decision-making discussed in the previous chapter. In the ADHD model discussed, almost all (90%) the explanations of behavior were uncovered in the cognitive model. Our client, a VP of pharmaco-economics in a leading pharmaceutical company, was surprised to see such powerful results in the cognitive model. He had not seen such a high level of explanation in any prior predictive modeling research in his thirty-five years in pharma. He asked how much of this was driven by the demographic data. We answered "None!" We had not included demographic data in the model. This was unheard of, and he asked why we didn't include the demographic data. We explained that the purpose of the model was a commercial application to behavior change: demographic variables are not something we can change, and as such they did not meet our criteria for inclusion in a behavior change model. Apparently, this was radical thinking! The VP asked that we re-run the cognitive model adding in the demographic data. With the new analysis, the power of the model increased from 90% to 90.01%: to be clear, that's one hundredth of one percent! The demographic data could not explain anything that the cognitive data hadn't already explained.

Perhaps the reason the VP had never seen such a powerful model before was that he had never used cognitive variables before. I believe this VP is not alone. It is well understood that demographic data are analyzed as surrogates for some other underlying factors that cause behavior. Insurance companies use this information very well to estimate costs and design tiered premiums. For example, red cars are involved in more car accidents than white cars, but it is not the "redness" that causes the accident. Rather, this is a surrogate for an underlying trait of a more risky driver. It is unfortunate that models built to predict costs of care are also labeled "predictive" when used to explain patient behavior. It is misleading to refer to them as "predictive" of behavior when they use surrogate markers and not the actual predictors of behavior that can be manipulated to create a change in behavior. There is nothing we can do about a patient's ethnicity or zip code to change his/her behavior. The real predictors—or at least 90% of them—are in the cognition that precedes the behavior. We need to remember that the surrogates (the color of the car, or the ethnicity of a patient) should never trump the real data (the cognitive factors) that are the true determinants of behavior. When this occurs in patient engagement strategy, it yields irrelevant communications to patients and does little to actually change behavior. The gaps in care remain, outcomes don't improve, and costs have been added, not removed.

An important feature of a model of how patients think is that not all factors are created equal. For example, in Figure 2 (page 64), the model shows that "Interpretation of disease etiology" is more than twice as powerful as "cognitive component #3."[ψ] This is important because if we only have one opportunity to communicate to this patient/caregiver, then we have to make sure we communicate that a biochemical interpretation is the basis for ADHD. If we fail in changing this single factor of how the patient/caregiver thinks, then it will be almost impossible to create the desired behavior change no matter what type of program the patient is in, how it is delivered, or when he/she is in it. Without the agents of change firmly embedded in the program, there is no scope to create the behavior change. Evaluation of the scope of the change agents should be done *before* committing resources to the program, even a pilot program.

KNOW THE ROI BEFORE YOU SPEND

A reliable cognitive model will also state how far the ROI can be driven by each cognitive factor. For example, for every dollar spent on communication of a stronger predictor, up to an 8:1 ROI can be expected, compared to communication of a weaker factor, where a 2:1 ROI might be expected. This is based on the total dollar return projected by closing the gap from baseline behavior to desired

---

[ψ] For proprietary reasons not all factors are revealed.

behavior (or more correctly, by closing 90% of the gap, per the model's power). Let's unpack this in a little more detail.

A publication of adherence rates in oncology showed that 26% of oncology patients who were prescribed oral treatment following surgery, radiation and/or chemotherapy were non-adherent to medication (defined as less than 80% Medication Possession Ratio [MPR] over 12 months).[52]

- The average MPR for this non-adherent group was 43%.
- These patients are valued at $22 per day (based on Wholesale Acquisition Costs [WAC] of the drug).
- So for 157 days of treatment (that is 43% of the year), they generate revenue of $3,454 at their current level of adherence.

A cognitive model was developed that explained the gaps between the adherent (>80% MPR) and the non-adherent (<80% MPR) patients. The model achieved 89% predictive power. Assuming reliable program design and execution, the baseline behavior should shift 89% of the way towards the goal. With a baseline behavior of 43% MPR (or 157 days of treatment), and a goal of 80% MPR (or 292 days of treatment), then the incremental days of treatment achievable from a model with 89% power are an additional 135 days of treatment.

The equation to estimate the model value per patient is thus:

$$Y = V[p(z-x)].$$

Where:

Y = $ Value of behavior change in the target segment,

V = Daily $ value per patient,

p = Model power,

z = Goal behavior,

x = Baseline behavior.

$$Y = \$22 \ [0.89 \ (292 \ days \ -157 \ days)];$$
$$Y = \$22 \ (0.89 \ X \ 135);$$
$$Y = \$22 \ X \ 120;$$
$$Y = \$2,640 \ incremental \ revenue \ per \ patient.$$

Knowing that 26% of patients are non-adherent *and* that they can be explained by the model, in a population of 100,000 patients, the total value of the model for the segment is:

$$Y = vns[x + p(z-x)].$$

Where n = the size of the population, and s = the proportion of patients not at goal.

The value of the model in this segment is:

$$Y = \$2,640 \ X \ 26,000 \ patients;$$
$$Y = \$68.6 \ million \ incremental \ revenue.$$

Thirteen factors in all explained this gap between the adherers and the non-adherers. As stated earlier, not all factors are created equal. Using the same formula as above, but substituting the individual contribution of each of the 13 factors for the total model power, the value of each factor can also be estimated.

$$\text{Value of Factor 1: } Y = vns[x + F1(z\text{-}x)],$$
$$\text{Value of Factor 2: } Y = vns[x + F2(z\text{-}x)],$$
$$\text{Etc.,}$$
$$\text{Value of Factor 13: } Y = vns[x + F13(z\text{-}x)],$$

Where F1 = Factor 1; F2 = Factor 2; etc., to F13 = Factor 13.

In this case, executing a truncated behavior change program based only on messaging around the top three factors (which account for 66% of the variance in behavior) across the business relevant segment of 26% of patients, in a sample of 100,000 cancer patients, yields a return of $51 million. Messaging around the single most powerful factor only (which accounts for 31% of the variance in behavior) yields a return of $24 million.

In another disease category, type 2 diabetes, a cognitive model was generated that differentiated between those who had controlled disease ($\leq$7.5% HbA1c mmol/moL) and those who did not (>7.5% HbA1c mmol/moL). **The savings in the total Medicare population who have diabetes was estimated at $3 billion per**

annum using only a portion (12%) of the total model parameters.[53]

Estimates of the effect sizes and how they translate to financial return on the investment should be run *before* programs are launched, even pilot programs. This is a simple check to assess if the model is even capable of returning the investment at all. Note that this is the *upside* potential and assumes that the development and execution of the program is of sufficient caliber to drive the conversion in cognition that the model states is required in order for the behavior change to occur.

COURSE CORRECTION #6:
DON'T WAIT UNTIL AFTER EXECUTION TO ESTIMATE THE ROI.
MAP THE PARAMETERS FOR CHANGE,
AND THEIR VALUE, *PRIOR* TO EXECUTION.

DEVELOPING MESSAGES THAT CHANGE THE COGNITIVE PROFILES

Actually carving out the communications that change behavior once a cognitive model is available is a simple task by comparison. Consider the ADHD example mentioned earlier. In the ADHD study, one of the strongest factors in explaining the difference between parents who sustained an extended pharmacological regimen for their child and those who terminated within 90 days was the parents' interpretation of disease etiology. Those parents who understood that there was a biochemical pathway behind their child's inattention maintained treatment. On the other hand, those who believed that ADHD was a behavioral condition terminated treatment within 90 days. Of course, the solution becomes very clear when we have identified a causal factor to the disengagement and can isolate those parents who have this barrier. In this case, the appropriate solution is to present to the parent some depiction of the biochemical nature of ADHD. It can be simple cartoon-type graphics, or more elaborate scientific information. In either case, the key is that the parent must believe that there is an underlying bio-chemical mechanism behind the disease. If they do not buy into that thinking, they will not maintain a pharmacological treatment plan. If they do embrace this thinking, and are influential in the home (see below), then they will be adherent.

Another distinguishing factor in those parents who terminated within 90 days was "Influence in the home." If one parent, say the mother, had bought into the biochemical nature of ADHD, but the other parent, say the father, had not, and the mother was unable to influence the father to adopt her way of thinking, then the treatment was not maintained. This area of exploration, "family dynamic," was included in the research because literature suggests that more than one person often contributes to healthcare decisions made on behalf of another (e.g., child or aging parent). We needed to know to what extent one parent can make a unilateral decision to introduce prescription medication to a child. We approached the decision-making process in the home from several angles. A series of questions was included in the survey to assess decision-making, not just in healthcare, but more broadly. Interestingly, one of the best discriminators for assessing this dynamic was the following question: "If you wanted to go to France on your holidays and your partner wanted to go to Italy, where would you end up going?" In fact, when compared to the question "Do you intend to continue treating your child with prescription medication for ADHD," the "holiday" question was actually a *stronger* predictor of adherence to medication. Now when we look across the entire predictive model, it is evident why the holiday question is a better predictor. The mother was very well aware of the biochemical nature of ADHD (or had been newly convinced of this in the physician's office), she understood that she could not manage her child's behavior through discipline alone, and she intended to continue treating her child with prescription medication because this made sense to her. Her mindset is that the child is sick, or at least has a condition that is impacting him at a biochemical level, and she needs prescription medication to rebalance him. She knows behavioral strategies alone are insufficient. Meanwhile, the father has a different mindset. He may not see his child as having a biochemical condition—after all, the child has no overt biological symptoms; he is not "sick"—and therefore does not need medication. Perhaps he agrees with the statement that the child's behavior can be managed with discipline alone. If the husband has a strong voice in decision-making and the mother cannot convince him sufficiently (as evidenced by the holiday question), then even though she may have bought into pharmacological treatment, her decision is overruled at home. Hence why a question about where they go on holiday predicts what the mother will do better than her intention to continue treatment. The importance of accounting for all (or most) of the factors is shown in this example. Had the model captured only half the factors, say omitting the "Influence in the home" factor, the program would fail to deliver the anticipated results through lack of overall efficacy.

Smoking cessation—success versus failure

Let's look at another important treatment category—smoking cessation. This particular health challenge incurs a high rate of failure in behavior change programs. What can be done to improve the success rates here for smokers and secure a positive return on investment for program providers? We will look at how to wrap a scientific theory of behavior around the decision to continue smoking or to quit. We will use the Health Belief Model (HBM) to understand the internal decision-making process of smoking (and cessation) and present what a solution to support smoking cessation might look like. Note, we have not brought this application of the HBM in smoking cessation into quantitative testing. The purpose of this illustration is to show how communication content can be developed from a backdrop of a theoretical approach to cognition and behavior. A model would need to be built to test these assumptions. Nonetheless, assume for now that any quantitative statics would support the HBM as an approach to smoking cessation! According to the Health Belief Model, whether consciously or subconsciously, our health behaviors are the result of how we project the *value* and the *downsides* of the healthy behavior, against the *value* and the *downsides* of the unhealthy behavior.

Applied to smoking cessation, the model might look something like this:

Table 4: A Health Belief Model approach to smoking cessation

	Benefits	**Downsides**
Smoking	A. I enjoy it My way to relax It's who I am	B. Poor health Future risks Smell/fumes annoy others Costly
Quitting	C. Save money Fresh breath Longer life with family Happy spouse	D. Cravings Jitters Fidgety hands Feel miserable

Smokers actually enjoy smoking. They find it relaxing and are comfortable with being smokers; it has become part of their identity and they are ok with that. They are well attuned to these benefits of smoking (see quadrant A in Table 4). As healthcare professionals, we might not want to acknowledge that there are real benefits to smoking, but to be relevant to the smoker, we must consider them. And we must provide a workable solution around these benefits in order to effect the change. Smokers do not relish the thought of quitting nearly as much as healthcare professionals! Quitting does come with downsides including cravings, the jitters, and smokers generally feeling miserable (see quadrant D). The majority of health campaigns put out by government, behavior change vendors, employers, health plans and pharmaceutical companies aim to deter the smoker by communicating the dangers of smoking (quadrant B) and the benefits of quitting (quadrant C). The vast majority of smokers know and believe that smoking is harmful to their health, so messaging around the dangers of smoking doesn't give them new information, and therefore will do little to change their behavior.

The smoker and the behavior change provider have vastly different vantage points, so the dialogue is off-balance and there is a disconnect. As a result, smoking cessation programs that present half the required information—the benefits of quitting (quadrant C) and the downsides of smoking (quadrant B)—are unpersuasive and irrelevant against the smokers' internalized value system, which is hinged upon the benefits of smoking and downsides of quitting (quadrants A & D). The smoker's concept of smoking, and the reason why he/she keeps smoking, has largely been left unchallenged by the "behavior change" communications.

Instead, to increase the relevance and the chances of success, the focus of communication ought to be on quadrants A & D. This is where the smoker is stuck in his/her own thinking. For example, challenging the benefits of smoking could include questions such as "Is smoking *really* you?" "Who/what started you smoking?" "Was that your decision?" "Did it feel 'right' then?" "When did it start to feel right?" "Is it right?" Equally, reframing the downsides to quitting could include counseling with coping mechanisms and alternative behaviors the smoker can get involved in when the urge strikes (go for a run, chew gum). This is where the creative agencies get creative and leave the scientists behind!

In summary, a scientifically based intervention that uses the Health Belief Model as its theoretical framework would include balanced messaging on *all four* components of persuasion, thereby actually increasing the relevance of the dialogue on the benefits of the smoking and downsides of the quitting (quadrants A & D), which are the real cognitive barriers that the smoker is struggling to shift. It would involve a persuasion to minimize these components of the thinking, as well as moderating a focus on the benefits of quitting and downsides of smoking. This provides a (i) comprehensive and (ii) relevant view of smoking that the smoker identifies with and can then use to re-balance his/her decision, thus raising the probability of successful cessation.

~   ~   ~

In developing multiple models of healthcare decision-making over the years, the strength of the model, and its ability to shape behavior change, is directly related to the robustness of the theory of behavior that the model captures. The strength of the model is not related to the amount of claims data, demographic data, or other purchasing type data. For example, in a breast cancer model, when looking at a single theory of behavior applied to medication adherence, 31% of the variance was explained across a sample of over one thousand women with breast cancer. When two theories of behavior were included, the variance explained rose to over 55%, and with three theories of behavior, a total of 66% of the variance in the patient's decision to adhere to medication or abandon treatment was explained. The model did not include any demographic data.

A NOTE ON EXPERIMENTATION

Let me put out a caution on the "experimental" approach to behavior change programs. A common approach to population health management today for many large companies is to pilot multiple programs for behavior change, as many as they can fund, and see which works best (if any works at all). Almost never do these programs have a *pre-identified* set of moderators of behavior at the crux of the change process being designed. They are then piloted on small samples and determined to be a success or failure only *after* the investment, when the results are in. With programs costing anywhere from half a million dollars to tens of millions of dollars each, this becomes a very expensive and inefficient approach. The equivalent in disease management would be a physician prescribing a treatment without first diagnosing the problem—just to see if it could be something a statin might help! Experimentation with options is valuable, but there needs to be a rational process behind choosing which programs to experiment with and how. A diligent use of resources involves assessing the odds that the investment will be worthwhile *prior* to making the investment, not after the fact when the money is lost.

To summarize, science-based interventions are those that:

(i)   Rely on the principles of the scientific method in their investigation;

(ii) Have a validated, peer-reviewed theoretical explanation of the behavior being changed, and;

(iii) Present a clear demarcation of how, and in whom, the behavior can be changed. That is, they have a pre-specified Mechanism of Action (MOA).

By this definition, science-based interventions are not currently used in healthcare—at least in terms of patient engagement or wellness solutions. How do you know, for example, whether a behavior change program will deliver against its objectives or not? How do you know if you are pursuing a red herring or whether you truly have something of substance? How can you know this *before* you invest millions of dollars in a program? Just as with drug development, a strong scientifically based platform is required as a basis for effective patient management strategies. Anything less will simply fail to generate significant and sustainable impact on outcomes at a patient or population level. Hindsight is 20/20—with a structured platform for patient-centric strategy, foresight can be too!

CHAPTER 7: IDENTIFYING THE HIGH-RISK SEGMENTS —THE RIGHT PATIENTS

It is important to keep in mind the two overarching reasons why patient support programs exist and why we invest billions of dollars in wellness and behavior change programs. First, we want to create healthier people (patients, employees, members, population); and second, we want to reduce the costs of care. With that in mind, the focus of our resource allocation efforts ought to be on those segments that are the driving force behind poor health and high costs. Unfortunately, the vast majority of healthcare stakeholders today (and that probably includes your company), are not actually doing this. Instead, "high-risk" segments that are the focus of behavior change programs are traditionally defined by one of two methods: (1) actuarial models based on patients' past behavior and demographics, or; (2) personality types. These methods are very far removed from the real business objective of actually reducing the costs of care by changing health behavior and, subsequently, make it very difficult to translate the benefit of the programs into measurable impact. The business goal needs to remain front and center, and it must inform the segments we select and focus on. Let's clear up some of the misunderstanding in current targeting approaches before discussing how *business objectives* can determine the basis of resource allocation, and thus, the targets for behavior change programs.

ACTUARIAL MODELS AS A BASIS OF RESOURCE ALLOCATION

Past behavior is a great predictor of future behavior only when the environment is controlled and unchanging, behavioral repertoire is limited, and cognitive prowess is capped at a fairly rudimentary level. For more complex behavior, it is a gross over-simplification of the complexity of decision-making to assume the status quo prevails, and in *all* cases where the estimated behavior is one of change, this assumption will yield the incorrect prediction. Consider a patient, Mrs. Brown, who has a claims history of being 50% adherent to her medication for depression. She receives a new diagnosis of diabetes. The model is run, and using her depression adherence rate as an input, she is predicted to be high-risk in diabetes since this insurer's model suggests that diabetes patients who consume less than 50% of their medication cannot maintain controlled HbA1c. Her annual cost of care at $11,700 is projected to escalate to $20,700 over the next three years.

There are several reasons why this "prediction" is not warranted. Are we to assume that there is no differentiable value between the treatment of diabetes and the treatment of depression? Are we to assume that Mrs. Brown has an equal perception of the threat of diabetes and the threat of depression? Are we also to assume that the reasons why she might fail to consume her diabetes medications are the very same as the reasons why she is currently non-adherent to her depression medications? What if a life-threatening disease such as breast cancer were to appear on Mrs. Brown's case file? Would the prediction of her perceived value of treatment for cancer be imputed from her depression medication consumption? Is every disease experience the same? Is every product created equal? From a marketing or branding perspective, what does this type of modeling even mean? It seems counter-intuitive to the fundamentals of conventional marketing to suggest that the value proposition of Mrs. Brown's diabetes medication is equal to the value proposition of her depression medication or breast cancer medication! Couldn't she have radically different perspectives and engagement patterns across her various diseases? Even if she were 50% adherent to treatments for two different diseases, it could be for very different reasons. We have already seen in the earlier case studies of ADHD and oncology that different factors underlie the decision (e.g., misinterpretation of etiology of disease is a major factor of non-adherence to ADHD treatments; it is meaningless for predicting adherence to breast-cancer treatments). Imputing a patient's engagement level using claims modeling is an over-extension of the application of actuarial data. When actuarial models are misapplied in this way, they create an unfortunate shift in the focus away from the true risk patients.

In fact, data suggests that these models actually miss 46% of real risk patients, and more remarkably, they create wastage of up to 66% in directing resources towards patients who are actually low risk when evaluated from a perspective of their ability to effectively self-manage! That is, the majority of the "high-risk" segments do not need any additional support beyond their clinical treatment in order to achieve their health goals, yet they are consuming 66% of patient support or wellness program spend! This has created billions of dollars in wasted resources, as misdiagnosed targets form the majority of intervention participants.

Let's look at the financial implications of using actuarial models to segment patients for support programs. We will assume an 80/20 split to conform with the convention of 20% of patients driving 80% of costs, and we will compare a traditional claims-based segmentation with a cognitive-based segmentation approach. With a business objective of isolating the 20% of cases that are driving costs, if we had perfect prediction, our segmentation of risk would look like the chart in Figure 3 below.

(a) Optimal resource allocation

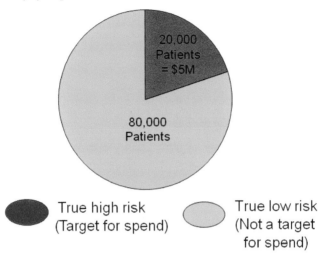

Figure 3: Segmentation of high and low risk with perfect prediction

Obviously in real world statistics/predictions, some level of error is to be accepted. But to illustrate, when there is no error in sorting out the high risk from the low risk (that is, all high risk have been successfully detected and no low risk have been misclassified as high risk), our perfect segmentations look like Figure 3 above. Figure 4 below shows how current claims-based models define these same high-risk and low-risk cases. This is a real world scenario based on current standards of predictive models used in healthcare.

(b) Current Claims-based spend

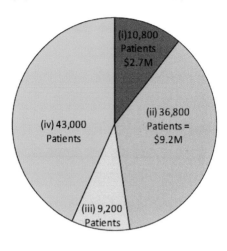

True high risk   True low risk
False high Risk   False low risk

Figure 4: Segmentation of high and low risk with claims-based prediction.

With this approach, there is significant error in misclassifying low-risk patients as high risk. In fact, of the total segment identified as high risk, two-thirds of them are not high risk at all (i.e., segment ii). If the high-risk cases are being identified for the purpose of resource allocation, this approach yields significant wastage. At an additional spend of, say, $250 for patient wellness support (e.g., telecoaching & incentives), the wastage is $9.2 million per annum on a total base of 100,000 patients. Compare this to Figure 5, which illustrates predictions based on cognitive profiling. Using the cognitive-based approach, the 66% wastage is practically eliminated, being reduced to 3%, an acceptable error rate. This recoups $9 million of the wasted $9.2 million. Furthermore, a higher proportion of the true high-risk cases are identified, creating a broader reach within the real target group—those patients who will generate 80% of the cost. In all, with the wider detection of real high-risk patients/employees, coupled with the reduction in wastage from false high risk, a net 55% reduction in the costs of outreach are achieved from the cognitive approach compared to standard claims-based approaches.

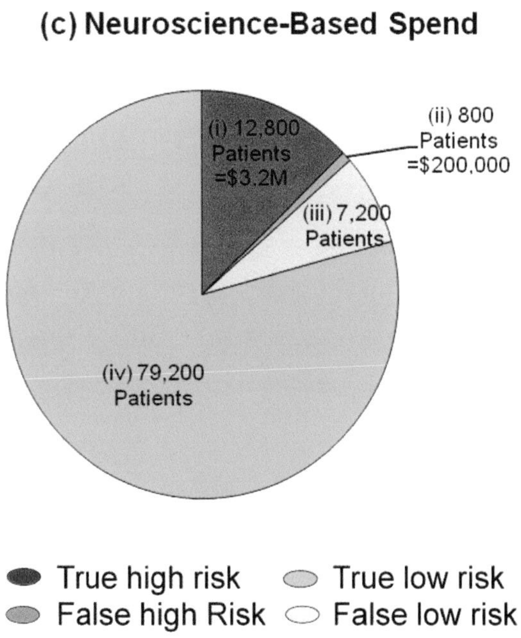

(c) Neuroscience-Based Spend

Figure 5: Segmentation of high and low risk with cognitive-profiling prediction.

PERSONALITY TYPES AS A BASIS OF RESOURCE
ALLOCATION

Another common approach in engagement strategy and wellness programs is to segment patients according to health personality types. At one end of the spectrum might be the "actively engaged," and at the other end might be the "aloof and disinterested." Whatever labels are used for these segments, solutions are then generated, for example, speaking positive "job well done" messages to the engaged. More importantly, though, a dilemma arises: are the "aloof and disinterested" to be persuaded to become more engaged, or are they to be left alone until some other time when they might become interested? Consider, for example, the Prochaska Stages of Change or Transtheoretical Model.[54] This model states that there are five types of patients aligned on a spectrum based on their willingness or readiness to make changes. At the lower end of the spectrum we have those who are not ready to change. They are said to be "Pre-contemplative;" they are not even *thinking* about making a change. The next level is "Contemplative," consisting of those who are beginning to consider that changes might be necessary. We move through the stages of "Preparation" and "Action" to the other end of the spectrum to those who are in a stage of "Maintenance."

According to this model, patients in the lower segments, the "Pre-contemplative" and "Contemplative" stages, are selected *out* for service provision and the more eager segments of "Action" and "Maintenance" are selected *in* for service provision. The very faulty and unscientific explanation given by Prochaska for this targeting is that the "Pre-contemplative" and "Contemplative" segments are not "ready" for change. From a behavior change perspective, not to mention an ethical perspective, it is precisely these patients who require additional support. Any model with integrity should be able to explain (i) *why* these patients are stuck in a "Pre-contemplative' state, and; (ii) *what*, exactly, needs to be done in order to support them so they can actively manage their healthcare and achieve their health goals. **Is that not the whole point of behavior *change* programs—to support behavior change in those who cannot change themselves?** These segments that are excluded from additional support services include the bottom 20% of patients who are driving 80% of the costs of healthcare and they need help! If providers of behavior change and wellness "solutions" truly understood the nature of the behavior being changed, they would not shy away from these needy segments. Indeed, they would target their programs specifically to those who actually need help, that is, the "Pre-contemplative" and "Contemplative" segments—not rule them out! Ψ

Rejecting these lower performing segments as not appropriate for change interventions is a cruel misfortune of an apathetic attempt to excuse the inability to drive a positive change where the change is

_____

Ψ The author is not referring the *physician* practice of screening out the sickest patients. Of course physicians treat all patients regardless of segment type. Rather the author is referring to the practice of health plans, pharmaceutical companies and vendors of support services for patients, who typically screen out patients who are difficult to change.

needed most. This is a disservice to a healthcare system struggling to improve outcomes and reduce costs of care as it continues to fuel the cycle of "increased costs-decreased outcomes" that has baffled the industry over the past decades. **To screen _out_ these people is entirely at odds with patient engagement as a strategy to improve outcomes and the cost of care.**

Moreover, advocating a strategy of providing costly support services to those who are already predisposed to manage healthy behavior in and of themselves is, quite literally, a waste of resources. This type of approach to patient care presents, at best, a scapegoat for checking-the-box of service provision, and, at worst, an ethical dilemma in the withholding of service to those who need it most. In fact, risk stratification to weed _out_ the sickest patients goes against the whole philosophy of healthcare delivery. It is not the healthy who need a physician, but the sick.[55]

Getting back to the business objective of population management and costs of care, in order to create an impact, our limited resources should be directed towards the harder-to-manage cases, the 20% of patients/employees who cannot manage their health by themselves. It is precisely these patients who would benefit from the investment, not to mention yield the largest return on the investment (ROI). But this is not happening in the healthcare market today. Why is that? Importantly, it is not because these tough patients cannot change. It is because a scientific platform for behavior change does not exist within the predominant models such as the Prochaska model of change,[56] or Patient Activation Measure (PAM).[57] These models cannot explain why patients are stuck in the "Pre-contemplative" or "Contemplative" segments, and so structuring a program to these segments would not actually create any change in behavior (and potentially embarrass the seller of the program)! If the model could explain the reasons behind disengagement, then the appropriate needy and costly segments ("Pre-contemplative" and "Contemplative") would be targeted for interventions to change their behavior. The results of this approach would be significant savings (66%) from not spending on already engaged patients, and a course correction by the bottom 20% of patients who are the most needy and costly (driving 80% of the costs of care). This would create a meaningful impact on outcomes, and yield even further cost savings from diverting predictable health complications in the high-cost segment.

COURSE CORRECTION #7:
PROCHASKA OR PAM DON'T IMPACT POPULATION OUTCOMES.
THE FOCUS MUST BE ON THE SICKEST 20%
WHO DRIVE 80% OF THE COSTS.

According to United Healthcare, the average cost of a patient
diagnosed with type 2 diabetes without complications is $7,800 per
annum.[58] Unfortunately, 17% of patients without complications will
escalate to severe diabetes[59] costing $20,700 per annum.[60] The value
of patient management strategy lies in detecting this 17% of patients
before they experience disease complications and reach the higher
bounds of costs of care. Therefore the business imperative operates
on how we isolate these 17% of patients early enough to direct them
away from their predictable future and secure more moderate
outcomes for them.

Earlier in Chapter 6, the financial ROI equation for behavior change
programs was illustrated. The return was estimated based on
increasing the suboptimal adherence rate from a baseline of 43%
Medication Possession Ratio (MPR) to a goal of 80% MPR (or
more accurately, towards 89% of that goal, or 76% MPR) in a
relatively small segment of 26,000 patients (i.e., the 26% of patients
who have an MPR <80%). In that example, the value of the
behavior change program in the business relevant segment was
estimated at $68.6 million incremental revenue for a pharmaceutical
manufacturer.

Let's have a look at how this ROI changes when we let fear of
failure shift the focus away from this tougher 26% of cases, and

place it on the easier, more engaged, segments. Now instead of taking the business relevant segment of the bottom 26% of poor adherers (i.e., those driving the costs), targets are selected from "Action" and "Maintenance" segments of patients who are 70% to 80% adherent. Our baseline of 43% consumption has now been reset to a new baseline of 75% consumption. Obviously, the opportunity to maximize the ROI has been removed—not a good starting place! Assuming the goal is still 80% consumption, we now have a significantly truncated upside potential of a mere 5%. The model can deliver 89% of the way to closing this gap of 5% MPR (to 4.5% MPR). That's sixteen extra days of therapy versus one hundred twenty extra days of therapy that is the real upside available to the business when focusing on the lower performing segment. Substituting these estimates into the same ROI model in Chapter 6 looks like this:

- Wholesale Acquisition Cost (WAC) of $22 per day;
- Incremental revenue per patient: $22 X 16 days = $352.

This scarcely covers the costs of providing additional support materials to the patient and has little impact, if any, on population health, and consequently, on reducing the costs of care.

Realizing a profitable return on investment in patient management strategy requires due diligence to the fundamentals of patient behavior. Fortunately, significant advances have been made in the past two decades in understanding complex behavior, much of which can be applied to patient decision-making. Enough, in fact, that even small accommodations that directly touch the cognitive system can generate significant impact on health behavior. Maladaptive health behavior can now be explained in definable scientific terms, profiled, moderated, and measured. Furthermore, with appropriate understanding, patients can be taught to self-manage and self-motivate to achieve desired health outcomes despite the requirements of planning, monitoring, course-correction and overcoming temptations before they become complicated and costly.

If the industry is to make a significant impact on health outcomes at a population level and the costs of care, then efforts MUST be re-directed towards the 20% of patients who generate 80% of the costs of care. Avoiding this segment will (a) thwart efforts to reduce costs of care (80% of the driving force is left untouched), and (b) blockade impact on outcomes at a population level (the sickest are not getting better). [Ψ] From both a cost and population health perspective, it is precisely these toughest to manage cases that require intervention. A robust science-based approach can, and should, be at the core of patient engagement strategy to achieve that end. After the appropriate patients have been accurately diagnosed for risk of disengagement (that is, those who cannot self-manage without support), it is important to align them with an intervention

[Ψ] The author is referring to health plans, pharmaceutical companies, and vendors who provide patient support materials, tele-coaching etc needing to shift their focus, not physician practices, where of course all segments receive appropriate treatment recommendations, regardless of segment.

that specifically maps to their pathway of thinking. This is the topic of the next chapter.

COURSE CORRECTION #8:
CURRENT PROGRAMS TARGET HEALTHY SECTORS.
BUT BEHAVIOR CHANGE MUST OCCUR IN THE SICKEST SECTORS
TO IMPACT POPULATION HEALTH AND COSTS.

CHAPTER 8: THE RIGHT PATIENT IN THE RIGHT
INTERVENTION—THE RIGHT ALIGNMENT

Many healthcare stakeholders (pharmaceutical companies, insurers, large employer groups) have allocated significant budget to a variety of health and wellness programs over the years. The experience of positive impact in population or employee health, however, is still a rarity. A common explanation for the lack of impact is that the "wrong" patients must be in the "wrong" interventions. So patients are shuffled around and the data reanalyzed. This trial-and-error approach consumes significant resources, but the impact on health remains negligible, and the connection of the right patients to the right programs seems illusive.

How can we take a more deliberate strategic approach to patient engagement and resource allocation? Again, here we can learn from our physician colleagues. They follow a simple process in which they make a formal diagnosis based on a set of markers and then select the appropriate treatment. The success in the physical arena is due to scientific pathways of disease having been identified, the availability of diagnostic tools to assess patients, and the availability of treatment options designed to specific disease pathways. There is no need for costly and inefficient trial-and-error approaches for many diseases. Alignment of the correct treatment to the diagnosis should be no more difficult in patient engagement than it is in the treatment of hyperlipidemia or asthma.

EMBEDDING A SCIENTIFIC MODEL WITHIN THE BUSINESS STRATEGY

With a scientific model of the mechanism of action behind healthcare decision-making and tools for profiling the cognition of individuals, we can diagnose the real targets (patients/employees) for intervention, *and* prioritize the change factors to be moderated in order to create healthy behavior. Chapter 7 outlined how to define business relevant patients for targeting. This chapter outlines how to align these business relevant segments to the appropriate interventions.

Let's look at an example within breast cancer. In this example, a pharmaceutical company wanted to improve adherence rates to aromatase inhibitors for breast cancer. A commonly accepted threshold for "good" adherence is 80% Medication Possession Ratio

(MPR). That is, across a one-year period, if a patient consumes (or more accurately, has been dispensed) 80% of a year's supply, then he/she is considered "adherent."

In collaborative work with Harvard Medical School, we analyzed national adherence data and found that 26% of patients with early stage breast cancer were non-adherent to adjuvant therapy (i.e., oral therapy post surgery, radiation, and/or chemotherapy) within the first year of treatment.[61] While an improved adherence rate overall was attractive for the pharmaceutical company sponsoring the research, the focus of the adherence effort was not on the majority segment—the 74% of patients who were above 80% adherent. Rather, it was argued that, strategically, the bottom 26% of patients would provide the focus for intervention. The 74% of patients in the "good" adherer segment were already being well protected in their fight against a recurrence of breast cancer. It was the lower segment of 26% of patients who needed the additional protection. And secondly, the upside potential for the business was very small in the majority group, who were already over 80% adherent to their medication. The focus was to be on improving adherence in the 26% of patients who were not currently at the goal. Further analysis showed that the baseline adherence rate in this target group was an average MPR of 43%. That is, they consumed an average of 43% of their recommended medication within the first year of treatment—a significant shortfall. The business objective was stated as: To decrease the proportion of patients who are suboptimally adherent to medication (<80% MPR) within the first year of adjuvant therapy. A strategy guide aligned to this business objective is presented in Figure 6.

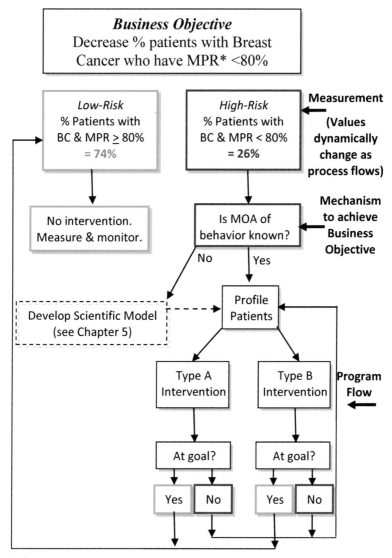

*MPR = Medication Possession Ratio (% days with treatment)

Figure 6: Strategy guide for scientific approach to oncology patient management programs.

So now that we have a business objective, and a strategic path to achieve that, let's take a tactical approach to securing the pull-through to deliver upon this objective.

To make the pull-through of strategy secure and achieve the business objective, a scientific model of adherence within oncology was developed. Data from nationally representative research confirmed several factors that explained the difference between the thought processes of the lower-end patients (averaging 43% consumption) and the higher-end patients (over 80% consumption). The research also included the development of a diagnostic tool that could provide cognitive profiles of patients with breast cancer. With this diagnostic, we could see who had a profile that predicted a solid adherence to her treatment regimen, and who did not (and why). Those who profiled as having a predisposition to disengage were recruited into an intervention. The tool extracted approximately 26% of patients. This was a strategic decision to reflect the business objective of homing in on those patients who were less than 80% adherent to their recommended therapy—which we knew was 26% of the breast cancer population. Figure 7 presents an example of a scientific model and how to wrap a strategic approach around a scientific platform for applied healthcare improvement.

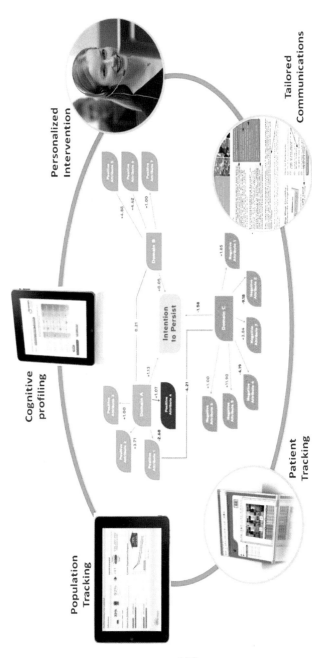

Figure 7: Graphic representation of a scientific model at the core of the process for identification, intervention and measurement in evidence-based patient-centric care.

Using this model, it became clear what differentiated the engaged from the disengaged and how we could profile or "diagnose" a patient's risk profile. For example, patients who were new to therapy were profiled around their "fight" versus "apathetic" stances regarding cancer. Those who profiled as "apathetic" were taught how to take a stronger stance in the fight against cancer. This mapping also highlighted the appropriate solutions now that we understood the causal links behind their non-adherent mindsets. Careful coaching and communications around this message was crafted to generate a significant shift in their thinking, and drive them towards healthy behavior. This of course, delivers the positive ROI for an intervention that is clearly mapped with the right message to the right patient at the right time. There is no need for costly trial-and-error approaches when the pathways to cognition and behavior have already been clearly mapped out *a priori*.

It has been stated before, but is worth stating again—in the research, 98% of patients also complained that their medications were too costly. By definition, this cannot be considered a causal factor in behavior change because almost all people agree on it. We must focus only on those factors that *differentiate* our target of 26% of breast cancer patients who are suboptimally adherent to medication from the norm. Cost does not differentiate them. I restate this because this faulty thinking is so entrenched in marketing and has been misapplied into the realm of behavior change. Total market thinking is not relevant to behavior change—and in fact, runs counter to the underpinnings of causation, which is the pivot point for change in behavior. Significant savings can be garnered through not spending on communications and coaching around messages that are not relevant to how patients think.

The results showed a dramatic impact. Initially the MPR in the target group began to increase from its starting baseline of 43%. A significant proportion of patients climbed high enough to reach the goal of 80% MPR and thus the drove the impact on our key metric of reducing the percent of patients with a MPR of less than 80%. For the first time in over five years of executing an adherence strategy, the adherence metrics began to improve and the change was evident at a population level.

~   ~   ~

A few important things to note in this approach are:

1. The business objective informed the initial questions: "How does the target segment (the bottom 26% of patients) differ from the norm? And how can we close the gap between them?"
2. All the variables stemmed from peer-reviewed verifiable theories of behavior and decision-making—that is, they were valid scientific explanations of behavior.

3. The mathematical model accurately captured the spectrum of thinking and differentiated the target group from the norm.

4. All the factors were modifiable under a process referred to as "cognitive restructuring" and formed the basis of the pull-through in patient communications.

5. A small set of variables was able to present a profile of risk at the outset of treatment, thus allowing for early intervention.

6. The cognitive profiles did not exclude any patients as being beyond repair or not "ready" to change. On the contrary, they isolated these needy cases as precisely the patients who need support. That is, the *right* patients for the *right* interventions at the *right* times.

In summary, when pursuing a targeted approach to patient engagement and population health, target segments must be clearly defined by business relevant goals. There is no place in a business focused patient engagement strategy to use less relevant groupings such as personality types, readiness to change segments, or past adherent behavior. It is imperative to keep the concentrated effort on the business objective at hand. Additionally, the type of intervention the patient receives should be informed by his/her cognitive profile. A program that has been specifically designed to moderate the change factors particular to that patient's profile should be selected—Diagnose first; then treat accordingly. Finally, no patient should be considered "not viable" for intervention unless he/she is already at goal. **Those at the lower end of the spectrum of health can indeed be changed, and in fact, the biggest impact on population health and costs of healthcare occurs by shifting those who are farthest from the goal towards the goal.**

CHAPTER 9: MEASURING PROGRESS TO GOALS
—THE RIGHT ROI

In chapter 8, we discussed the importance of business objectives remaining front and center in the development of patient engagement and population health strategy. The business objective, stated in operational terms, is ultimately the metric that trumps all metrics. If the plan isn't delivering positive results to progress the business objective, then the plan needs reworking. In his book, *Business Process Improvement*, H. James Harrington, International Quality Advisor for Ernst & Young, states "*Measurement is the first step that leads to control and eventually to improvement. If you can't measure something, you can't understand it. If you can't understand it, you can't control it. If you can't control it, you can't improve it.*"[62]

Measurement is what validates or refutes whether what we are doing is working. It is the yardstick that states if we are achieving the results that will progress our internal business objectives and return value to our external customers. Metrics can be considered the bookends of strategy. Strategy begins by stating the business objective in measurable terms, and ends with a clear analysis as to whether the plan delivered its objective or not. For example, consider the earlier business objective of reducing the proportion of breast cancer patients who are not at the adherence goal of 80% MPR. Our key measurement answers the question, "Is the plan decreasing this segment of 26% of patients who are not at goal?" If it is, the plan should continue. If not, resources should be reallocated and the strategy, or the plan around it, should be reevaluated.

Measurements in healthcare can be as broad as population preventative measures, such as the percent of children receiving vaccinations; or more specific, such as the percent of diabetic patients with HbA1c less than 8% mmol/moL in a given healthcare plan. Regardless of the measurement, a few good practices implemented around metrics and analytics can help keep us on track in our own decision-making and accountability to the business, encouraging continued investment when the measured value is high, or conversely, highlighting that a redirection of resources is appropriate when the measured value appears low. This chapter aims to highlight some of the pitfalls in current measurements and warn how faulty measurement can lead to decisions to misdirect resources into avenues that, although they report a positive ROI, still fail to impact business objectives, such as population health or the value of care.

Typically, patient management programs are measured in ways that present an exaggerated ROI. To illustrate, as discussed earlier, the targets for intervention are typically patients who are in the highest one or two quartiles, while the hard to manage cases, the lower quartiles, are selected *out* of intervention. This is predicated on the faulty assumption that these lower quartiles are "not ready to change." From a measurement perspective by itself, this wouldn't be a problem if the patients in the intervention were compared to the same type of high-quartile targets in a control group. However, most support programs such as wellness coaching, smoking cessation programs, adherence programs, etc., take the higher quartiles into the intervention, and then when the intervention is complete, compare them to a general sample that includes all comers—high and low quartiles.

The falseness of the ROI that is generated is twofold. First, the control group to which the targets are being compared includes the worst cases, which drag down the reported behavior in this group, rather than an appropriately matched group of high-quartile patients. And second, the high-quartile group that receives the intervention would have achieved the desired results anyway—even *without* intervention—since they were preselected on the basis of already having the mindset necessary for healthy engagement. Essentially, this is sandbagging the results.

Scenario 1—High Quartile Test Group Vs Average Control Group

Say we had 10,000 patients go through a patient support program to improve adherence to asthma treatment. A typical approach is to use a screening tool to segment personality or attitudinal types and then offer the higher segments (e.g., more motivated, more active, or ready for change) an opt-in to an intervention. These patients are provided with a program of telecoaching and their prescription activity is monitored. Results show that on average, patients in this intervention are filling about ten of their twelve monthly prescriptions over a year and so have a Medication Possession Ratio (MPR) of 83%.

In contrast, a control group is reported to have seven prescriptions over the year, for an MPR of 58%. This sounds like a very impressive and satisfactory difference between the intervention and control groups. So we might draw the conclusion that the program has earned the pharmaceutical company three additional prescriptions per person in the program. If the program costs $60 per person and it recouped three additional prescriptions per person valued at $180 (three months at $60 each), one might conclude that the program returned an impressive 3:1 ROI. A business decision might be made to expand the program to one hundred thousand patients for a cost of $6,000,000. A great deal with a volume discount might even be negotiated for one million patients capped at a cost of $30 million. This is illustrated below.

Scenario 1 Reported ROI

Test group = 10 Rx over 1 year;

Control group = 7 Rx over 1 year;

Reported incremental benefit = 3 Rx @ $60 = $180;

Program cost per patient = $60;

Reported ROI = 3:1;

Business decision = Scale up (1 million patients; negotiate $30 million deal).

This is a very typical approach to reporting the impact of behavior change and adherence programs in the healthcare industry. However, as mentioned above, the analysis contains two very serious flaws.

Scenario 2—High-Quartile Test Group Vs. High-Quartile Control

Let's see how the ROI changes when we correct these flaws and how the investment decision around the $30 million deal might change. We can take the same ten thousand patients and the same screening tool and put them into the same intervention. The first correction we'll make will be to compare these high-quartile patients with an appropriate control group —a high-quartile group that does not get the intervention. Now after the intervention, results show that the people in our test group are filling an average of ten of their twelve prescriptions over the year—that's an MPR of 83% — the same results as before. However, the control group, which is also high-quartile, is filling an average of 9.8 prescriptions a year—that's an MPR of 82%. The results don't seem so compelling when matched against an appropriate control group. At a cost of $60 per person and an incremental 0.2 prescriptions per person, that's returning a value of $12 (20% of $60 per full prescription). We now have a very different conclusion—the ROI is now a *negative* 2:1. Of course the business implication is significant. The $30 million-deal negotiated under Scenario 1 is not a wise investment after all. A small change in the analysis creates a stark shift in the business reality. This is illustrated below.

Scenario 2 Reported ROI

Test group = 10 Rx over 1 year;
Control group = 9.8 Rx over 1 year;
Reported incremental benefit = 0.2 Rx @ $60 = $12;
Program cost per patient = $60;
Reported ROI = -2:1;
Business decision = Terminate program (do not negotiate $30 million deal).

Unfortunately, a significant number of engagement and wellness solutions in today's market are analyzed in this mismatched manner. When personality or attitudinal or readiness-to-change methods are used as the basis of targeting, it typically focuses the resources on those who would have successfully managed their health anyway. Their performance is then analyzed against a general normative group. Since a primary objective of patient engagement and wellness programs is to improve health, as well as to lower the cost of care, it seems intuitive to place the emphasis for change on the segments that are struggling to maintain good engagement by themselves rather than the high-quartile group.

Scenario 3—Low Quartile Test Group Vs. Matched Control

Now we'll take this same scenario and look at how the ROI from our patient management efforts shifts when we focus our resources towards the other end of the spectrum—the lowest quartiles, who actually need additional support services. We take the same volume of patients, ten thousand, and screen them, but now we select in those at the lower end of the spectrum. This group of low quartiles has an average of five prescriptions across the year, that's an MPR of 42%. We deliver the intervention to the test group, withhold some as a matched control group, and the results show that the test group achieves seven prescriptions a year, that's an MPR of 58%. They are still short of the goal of 80% MPR and short of their high-quartile peers at 83% MPR. But compared to their matched control peers at 42% MPR, they have shown significant improvement (and perhaps will continue to improve into the next year). Now let's look at the ROI. This test group is returning two additional prescriptions valued at $120 per person (2 X $60) and yields a 2:1 ROI. Potentially they could improve by three, four, or more, up to a total available upside of seven additional prescriptions from their starting point of five prescriptions over a one-year period. This is illustrated below.

Scenario 3 Reported ROI

Test group = 7 Rx over 1 year;

Control group = 5 Rx over 1 year;

Reported incremental benefit = 2 Rx @ $60 = $120;

Program cost per patient = $60;

Reported ROI = 2:1;

Business decision = Invest more to scale up.

These three scenarios all use the same intervention and the same results. The examples above reveal how widely varying, and misleading, reports can be—enough to swing a "Go" decision to a "No go." The conclusions are:

1. When high-quartile patients are compared to an inappropriate control group, a falsely elevated ROI of 3:1 is reported—this has zero impact on the business objective.

2. When high-quartile patients are compared to their appropriate controls, the ROI is a negative 2:1–this has a negative impact on the business objective.

3. When the right patients (lower quartiles) are compared to their matched controls, a reliable 2:1 ROI is reported (with significantly more upside potential available)–this has a significant positive impact on the business objective.

COURSE CORRECTION #9:
KNOW YOUR NUMBERS.
ROI'S ARE NOT ALWAYS WHAT THEY SEEM
HENCE THE FLAT EFFECT ON POPULATION HEALTH.

~ ~ ~

A CONCLUSIVE APPROACH FOR MEASUREMENT

Obviously, when an ROI is falsely elevated, the impact does not follow through to real change in health behavior or a real impact on the business goal of providing better quality care under controlled costs. This is why, **despite the fact that many programs *report* a 3:1 ROI, there still has been no impact on population health over the past decade**. The results are misleading, inflated by skewed analyses. In contrast, a scientifically based approach, as in

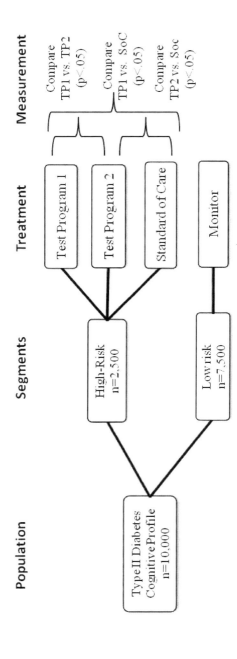

Figure 8: Measurement design for targeted impact in high-risk (low quartile) segments.

the practice of medicine, would target those who require intervention in order to effect the change we want to see in health outcomes—we diagnose to treat. When the right patients are compared to a *matched* control, the ROI is dramatic. Figure 8 below shows a measurement design with appropriate control group. In this design, two new programs are compared with the standard of care (the control group) for the same type of high-risk patients. High-risk patients are those in the lower quartiles (the bottom 25% to 50% of patients) who are driving the bulk of the cost in the healthcare system. With this design, there is no selective bias towards healthier people in the test group, the true targets are pulled into the intervention and like is compared with like.

Reliable measurement of behavior change includes: (i) *matching* the control group to the test group; (ii) taking *baseline* measures before the intervention; (iii) *random* allocation of subjects to Test versus Control segments; (iv) *measurement* (during and) at the end of the intervention to compare the Test group to the Control group. Fundamentally, any analysis must answer the following business questions unequivocally: "Are patients in the test group getting better or not?" and "Is the investment providing worthwhile return or not?"

As the appropriate high-risk group (low quartiles) flows through an intervention that is tailored to its cognitive profile, periodic testing should be conducted in order to assess the change relative to the baseline and relative to the control group. Several levels of measurement can, and should, be taken. In the clinical world we call these "endpoints." In patient engagement strategy we can adopt a similar rubric and also specify, *a priori,* what type of impact we expect at various endpoints. These various levels of measurement, or endpoints, range from very early reads in cognitive change to behavior change, outcomes impact, and ultimately the cost of care. Each of these endpoints provides unique insight as to how the business strategy is progressing. These are shown in Figure 9.

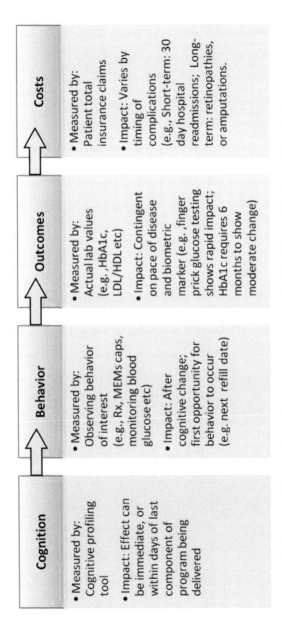

Cognition

- Measured by: Cognitive profiling tool
- Impact: Effect can be immediate, or within days of last component of program being delivered

Behavior

- Measured by: Observing behavior of interest (e.g., Rx, MEMs caps, monitoring blood glucose etc)
- Impact: After cognitive change; first opportunity for behavior to occur (e.g. next refill date)

Outcomes

- Measured by: Actual lab values (e.g., HbA1c, LDL/HDL etc)
- Impact: Contingent on pace of disease and biometric marker (e.g., finger prick glucose testing shows rapid impact; HbA1c requires 6 months to show moderate change)

Costs

- Measured by: Patient total insurance claims
- Impact: Varies by timing of complications (e.g., Short-term: 30 day hospital readmissions; Long-term: retinopathies, or amputations.

Figure 9: Progressive and contingent measurement plan for patient-centric strategy

It is important to note that these endpoints are: (i) *progressive*—the time to detect reliable change is longer as we move from the cognitive (on the left of Figure 9) to the ultimate endpoint of costs of care (on the right of Figure 9), and; (ii) *contingent upon one another*—forward progress from left-to-right is *not* possible without successfully creating the required impact on the preceding endpoint. The expected time to detect a measureable change depends on the level of change being measured. For example, a *cognitive* change can be seen as early as days or weeks into an intervention. The *behavior* change can be measured by actions such as filling the next month's supply of medication. The time to detect a meaningful change in *outcomes* can be short for acute conditions (e.g., ER visits within 30 days of surgery), or longer for chronic conditions (e.g., it takes at least 6 months to detect a 0.7% change in HbA1c). Finally, time to detect change in *cost* of care is the furthest out, as the financial consequences of disease control (or uncontrolled disease) take time to materialize and are also dependent on whether the disease is acute or chronic. For example, the costs of non-adherence to emergency room discharge instructions can be encountered within 30 days of discharge. In contrast, with a chronic condition such as diabetes, the cost impact may be longer term, as complications such as retinopathy or amputations may not occur for several years.

In addition to a fiscally responsible approach to intervention management, these early reads also offer a mechanism for quality control. Cognitions are predictable such that the scope for change is directly related to:

1. How many factors are behind the decision to behave/engage/quit;
2. How many of these factors are embedded in the patient engagement program, and;
3. How strong the communication is in hitting home the core messages.

If early available data on cognitive profiles suggests an engagement program is having little impact, then components of the intervention can be revamped to more powerful messaging depending on where the cognition is proving difficult to shift. For example, suppose a cognitive model showed that smokers who failed to quit did not have sufficient belief in the benefits of quitting but held strong beliefs in the benefits of smoking. Analysis of the cognitive change might reveal that the smoker's beliefs in the benefits of smoking were effectively challenged, but that the program failed to impact his/her interpretation of the benefits of quitting. In this case, the smoker will not be successful in his/her attempt to quit, since the program failed to moderate a major predictive variable. This can happen if too many extraneous or irrelevant messages have diluted the key messages required for change. In this case, new messaging that effectively challenges the benefits of smoking needs to be instilled in the program. Strong messaging that is pure to the causal factors of decision-making behind the behavior is critical in any behavior change program.

The cognitive change should be measured as an early indicator of the effectiveness of the patient engagement program. With successful impact at a cognitive level, the behavior change will follow in time, and the corollary is also true—failure to impact at a cognitive level means the behavior change will not follow.

In sum, **cognition precedes behavior**. That's worth repeating:

> ### COURSE CORRECTION #10:
> ### COGNITION PRECEDES BEHAVIOR.
> WITHOUT A CHANGE IN COGNITION,
> THERE IS NO CHANGE IN BEHAVIOR.

Figure 10 illustrates a design that incorporates these progressive and contingent endpoints into a pilot—one that compares two test arms to a matched control in high-risk targets.

The advantage of having different levels of measurement within the patient management initiative is that earlier reads from the cognitive

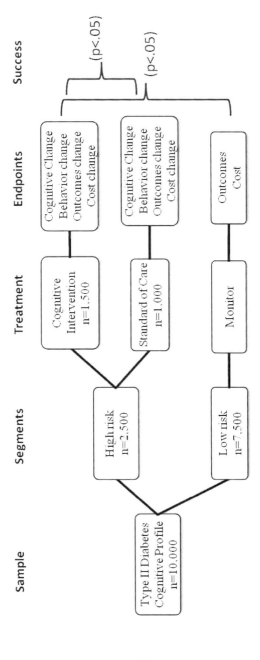

Figure 10: Comprehensive design for fiscally responsible patient engagement strategy

and behavior change can provide input into quality control in due time for course correction and reallocation of resources if necessary. Regardless of where the key business objective metric sits (e.g., progressing a health outcome, or reducing the cost of care), a fiscally responsible approach to patient engagement strategy and population health embeds early reads of potential success (or failure) into the plan. A comprehensive set of measures can track endpoints from cognitive change in specific segments through to the global impact on population health and costs of care. It also provides a vigilant mechanism to state the contingencies upon which successful achievement of the business goal is dependent.

PART III

CREATING MEASURABLE HEALTH AND WEALTH WITHIN THE US ECONOMY

CHAPTER 10: TRANSLATING PATIENT-CENTRICITY INTO POPULATION MANAGEMENT

A large focus of this book has been on patients' levels of engagement within the healthcare system. But to be clear, **the purpose of patient engagement is to support the effective delivery of interventions on a broad-enough scale to improve population health.** The focus on improved engagement is really part of a bigger strategic goal of improving health outcomes with enough vigor to create an impact at a population level. This is why *health outcomes* define how the scientific approach gets applied (Chapter 9). It is why *health outcomes* define what we do with patients we have profiled (Chapter 8). And it is why *health outcomes*, rather than surrogate markers such as household income, ethnicity, or personality segments, define the targets for intervention (Chapter 7). The further away any part of the process gets from the actual business goal of improved outcomes, the more our ability to reach that goal is stifled.

Population management is a popular theme in the healthcare system today. The 2010 enactment of the Patient Protection and Affordable Care Act (ACA) has resulted in the emergence of many new entities called Accountable Care Organizations (ACOs), in which accountability for health outcomes is defined and measured against goals for total populations. For example, the number of emergency room readmissions within 30 days across all cardiac surgery patients is a new metric of interest and one that can influence the level of reimbursement that practices or insurers receive from treating government-insured Medicare patients. Indeed, a single health plan can lose more than $100 million in reimbursement in failing to meet this one metric. Nationally, US healthcare spend is a staggering $3 trillion, 17.5% of GDP,[63] and it stands to climb higher as the population ages. It seems as if we have saturated our capacity for coping with and paying for ill health. Health plans, employers, and government can no longer afford the massive financial consequences of uncontrolled disease at a national level. The system has reached the breaking point. It has become more important than ever to translate patient-centric strategy into positive health outcomes at a population level.

To make an impact in population health, and reduce the national tally of healthcare costs for employers, health plans, and government, we need to be able to bring about substantial behavior change in individual patients and repeat the process efficiently. At the risk of oversimplifying, **population management is individual patient care on a large scale.** Populations are collections of groups, who are collections of individuals. There is nothing illusive, or gestalt, about populations; they are the sum of the individuals, nothing more and nothing less. This is good news, because when we have understood how to create significant change at an individual patient level, and have an efficient method for replicating the process on a broad scale, we have an effective strategy for population management. Essentially, to successfully translate patient-centric care into population health outcomes, the following three criteria are required: (1) identification; (2) intervention, and; (3) replication.

To impact health outcomes at a population level, we must:

1. *Accurately identify* the relatively small proportion of patients who currently restrain our ability to impact population health goals;
2. *Proactively intervene* in these high-risk cases before the mitigating factors impinge significantly on outcomes and costs, and;
3. *Efficiently replicate* the process across the targeted population.

This book has presented a comprehensive approach to the first two of these requirements including the initial scientific framework (Chapter 5); cognitive modeling (Chapter 6); diagnostic tool development (Chapter 7); intervention design (Chapter 8); matching profiled patients to their required intervention (Chapter 8); and business relevant measurement (Chapter 9). These components work synergistically. As the process of investment unfolds (see Figure 6, page 114), early analysis can inform whether continued investment is fruitful, or whether a reformulation of the intervention is required to drive the desired outcome (see Figure 9). The process is business relevant, predictable, self-correcting, fiscally responsible, and outcomes driven. Assuming we can execute such a comprehensive scientific strategy to support steps (i) and (ii) above, the challenge becomes replicating it enough to impact population health. Here's the simple formula for scale:

Replication Process + Access = Scale!

REPLICATION PROCESS

The starting point for constructing a process to replicate patient-centric strategy (or any other process) at a population level is defining the end goal. What impact on population health are we aiming to effect? When operating by a scientifically based strategy, decisions are made on an *a priori* basis of knowing *which* patients contribute stress on the healthcare system and *why*, and structuring patient-centric strategy *proactively* around these people *before* complications arise. This removes the trial-and-error approach that typically contributes further costs to an already strained system, and replaces it with a roadmap of how to navigate from A (unengaged patients) to B (scaled impact at a population level). A few examples of defining outcomes–driven end goals are presented below:

- To reduce the percent of patients with type 2 who have HbA1c > 9% mmol/moL;
- To reduce the number of ER admissions within thirty days of cardiac surgery;
- To increase the proportion of smokers who successfully quit over the next twelve months;
- To reduce the patients of patients with breast cancer who are sub-optimally adherent (< 80% MPR).

The flow chart in Figure 11 provides an example of a process for achieving the type 2 diabetes end goal. The business objective is stated as: *Reduce the proportion of patients with type 2 diabetes (T2D) with HbA1c > 9% mmol/moL.* This whole process supporting population management (segmentation, design, intervention, and measurement) is built around a precise business objective to improve a specific health outcome in a specific high-risk segment. As discussed earlier, with accurate profiling and alignment to a tailored intervention, positive patient-centric results are achieved. With increasing volumes of high-risk patients moving through this process, the scaled impact on population health and the costs of care become the natural outgrowth of the replication. This is referred to as the BPR process to population management: **B**usiness objective; **P**atient-centric; **R**eplication. The process streamlines the patient-

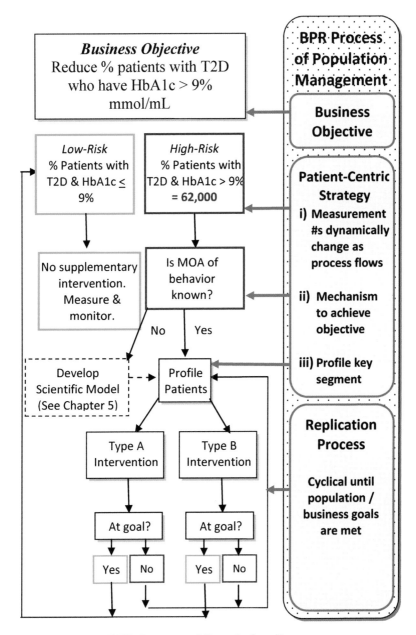

Figure 11: The BPR Process of Population Outcomes Management

centric activities around the business objective to deliver business relevant results.

The business objective, whatever it is, is what dictates the process for patient-centric efforts and, consequently, population health. It defines the "right patients" (e.g., diabetes patients with a HbA1c above 8% mmol/moL, or smokers, or whoever); it shapes the scientific modeling for behavior change (e.g., why do some smokers quit and others fail to quit?); and it states the measurement plan (e.g., how many successfully quit and is this enough?).

ACCESS—GETTING TO THE HEART OF THE MATTER

So with a robust platform for appropriate identification of true risk patients and aligned interventions, and a process plan from which to guide rollout, the challenge becomes effecting change in sufficient volumes to generate impact at a population level. How can we reach a sufficient number of patients to create an impact at a population level? This challenge is reported frequently by healthcare professionals, including insurers, pharmaceutical manufacturers, and service providers, as a barrier to effecting population outcomes. Let's unpack this a little. According to the Kaiser Family Foundation, almost 90% of the US population have access to healthcare through their employer, government, or private insurance.[64]

If 90% of the population have access to the healthcare system, wouldn't that mean that the healthcare system has access to 90% of the population? For example, every patient who has received a diagnosis of diabetes (or hypertension, or COPD, or had an ER visit for any other condition) has had at least one interaction with a healthcare provider. If not, he/she would not be on file as having a diagnosis or ER visit. Every patient who has filled a prescription has had at least one encounter with a pharmacist, either live, or via an automated system. Almost half (49%) the US population are insured by their employers,[65] which have frequent interaction with them (albeit on an "employee" basis rather than a "patient" basis). Even though this is a contractual relationship between the employer and the employee, the connectivity is there; the relationship exists. It's the same with government-insured patients; 32% of beneficiaries are covered by Medicare or Medicaid creating relationships where it is possible to interact.[32] Interaction with patients *is* happening and it is happening on a national scale. Access exists—and on many different levels at that, through employers, insurers, physicians, nurses, pharmacists, manufacturers, etc.

But *what* is happening during these interactions? In addition to providing health coverage and health services, such as diagnoses and treatment, what can be done within these existing interactions to generate the health outcomes we all want to see? Employers want to see their workforce in a healthier, more productive state; Medicare and Medicaid want to see their beneficiaries in better health and costing less; insurers want to see improved outcomes and reduced costs; pharmaceutical and device manufacturers want to see utilization of their products increase so they can realize their projected returns; and physicians (particularly those tied to Accountable Care Organizations) want to see their patients' outcomes improve. But do we want all these things badly enough?

MEGA-SHIFTS IN HEALTHCARE: THE REAL NATIONWIDE ISSUE

While the infrastructure may exist for interaction with patients, clearly something is missing. Replication on a national scale isn't happening. I do not believe the challenges are traditional scale or distribution issues. I believe the challenge in realizing significant improvements in population health sits closer to home—within our own walls of operation, and even within ourselves.

Adopting a scientific approach to population management requires mega-shifts across the span of the healthcare system. These are not quick fixes, but long-term reformulations of healthcare. They need to be embraced with urgency to allow us to achieve our goals for improved population health. Some are:

- *Applied Science:* It requires an extension of the bench from inside the laboratory to the field—into the environment where care is delivered, and into the home. It is insufficient to leave science in the laboratory, or in the physician's office. Science must permeate our patient engagement solutions to effect a significant and meaningful change in health.

- *Physicians:* It requires a reframing of the role of the physician to provide cognitive, as well as physical, diagnoses of their patients—assessments of the patients' totality to understand who they are, and the environment they live and work in, physically, socially, emotionally, and cognitively.

- *Interventions:* It requires a shift away from marketers and graphic designers as the central developers of support programs, and instead leverages researchers, scientists, and theory of behavior experts as the foundation for intervention design, just as in the treatment and management of other maladaptive conditions, such as depression, emotional breakdowns, and neuroses. We need to stop basic programs and, instead, cut deeply into the complex reality of how patients think.

- *Education:* It may even require a redrafting of the undergraduate and postgraduate curriculums surrounding the delivery and management of healthcare to accommodate the required changes noted above.

- *Accountability:* It requires more accountability than is required by health laws from every healthcare professional within the system; more accountability for what we do, why we do it, who we do it to, the results we measure, and the impact (or lack of) on health outcomes. We need to learn from our failures and build off our successes.

- *Purpose:* It requires a mind shift in how we, as healthcare professionals, conceive of healthcare, the purpose of the healthcare system, and our roles as professionals within it. This may, in fact, be one of the most difficult facets of the healthcare system to change.

A seriously broken system requires a serious overhaul at several system-wide levels. _We_ are the agents, as well as the *objects*, of change. And that is indeed a formidable barrier to scale!

Chapter 11: A Call to Action—A Redefinition of Healthcare And Our Roles Within It

If a single statement can capture the premise of healthcare, it may be Merriam-Webster's definition of the word: *"efforts made to maintain or restore health."*[66] That's a simple directive for any stakeholder in the business or practice of healthcare. It would seem from the decline in the health of the nation that we have fallen short of delivering on our basic premise.

The World Health Organization (WHO) suggests that *"contemporary perspectives on diabetes care accord a central role to patient self-care, or self-management."*[67] The same can be said of any disease—the patient's role is critical in achieving the desired outcome. Stakeholders are well aware of the consequences of poor patient engagement and many have deployed efforts to create more engaged patients who can effectively self-manage. Pharmaceutical companies, several pharmacy chains, insurers, and large employers have instituted programs to improve patient engagement. However, despite spending billions of dollars on patient support programs, we still have the same adherence rates we did in the 1970's[68] and the population generally is getting sicker, not healthier.

MULTI-CHANNEL DEPENDENCY

From an industry perspective, it can be difficult to ascertain the entities within the system that are ultimately responsible for improving health outcomes. Who, for example, is charged with informing patients about their diseases so they can effectively manage their health outside the clinic? Should physicians be held accountable since they have the training to select the appropriate treatments for their patients and make treatment recommendations to them? Newer models of pay-for-performance in Accountable Care Organizations (ACOs) impose some responsibility on physicians through shared financial controls/incentives. But can physicians monitor patients to the extent required to provide appropriate interventions when the patients show signs of disengagement? Perhaps the responsibility for achieving improved health outcomes should belong to pharmaceutical companies? The benefit/risk value equation that secures FDA approval for a drug and forms the basis for how it is promoted is based on levels of consumption in clinical trials (typically over 95%), not levels of consumption in the real world. Perhaps, in order to achieve this same benefit/risk outcome in the market place, a companion patient engagement strategy is required? Or perhaps the responsibility for achieving improved outcomes should belong to insurers? They can spot patients who are defaulting on recommended treatment plans long before other stakeholders, and they have a contract to provide care for patients—does that generate a responsibility? Perhaps achieving good outcomes is the patients' responsibility. Undoubtedly, they hold a central role, but can they get the support they need when they need it? Are they even aware that they need support? Can they recognize it before it's too late? Given that so much is at stake for every entity connected to healthcare (public and private), it is incumbent on each stakeholder to be an integral part of a more inter-connected patient management solution.

AN EYE ON THE PRIZE: LONG-TERM HEALTH AND WEALTH

Effectively and efficiently delivering healthcare requires multiple touch points to the patient, all of which have the potential for radical success *if*: (1) improved health outcomes are the common goal, and; (2) the long-term strategy is allowed to trump short-term wins. Table 5 outlines examples of short-term strategies for the various stakeholders in healthcare. It also presents a long-term strategy that could take its place. These are presented assuming a shared goal

Table 5: Short-Term versus Long-Term Strategies for Improved Health Outcomes

Stakeholder	Short-Term Strategy	Long-Term Strategy	Why Long Term wins
Insurer	Manage to annual budgets. Investment in future is constrained in tough economy; patient may switch to competitor in years to come eliminating return on long-term care.	Improved outcomes minimize future complications that are more costly than patient management solutions. Patients with better outcomes have higher satisfaction and retention.	Churn rates across different providers are comparable,[1] i.e., what goes around comes around. Reducing complications creates healthier, less costly patients.
Pharmaceutical & Device Manufacturer	Management looks for daily/weekly competitive gains in prescription transactions; shareholders look for short-term share value and growth.	Translating clinical efficacy into improved outcomes in the real world offers higher drug value and better risk/benefit profile. Value for payer customers. Builds trust.	Failure to replicate laboratory benefit in real world allows competitors to gain. [2] Outcomes-driven partners win contracts with payers.
Physician	Sicker patients return to the office for treatment maintaining a solid business flow.	Healthier patients require less time, allowing practices to grow their new patient bases. Healthier patients increase ratings and shared savings.	The demands of a sick practice compromise ability to cultivate growth of new patients thus challenging the sustainability of the practice.

Stakeholder	Short-Term Strategy	Long-Term Strategy	Why Long Term wins
Patient	A busy life and competing priorities lead to sporadic daily management of sickness when it occurs.	Incremental steps today help avoid significant complications later, which will compromise lifestyle and productivity	A healthy lifestyle enables more effective daily living and ability to plan, achieve, and enjoy, life goals.
Pharmacist	Educating patients on medication takes time from running the business and adds administrative burden.	Focusing on relationship building through care of customers creates sustainable base and higher referral growth.	A satisfied customer is a loyal customer to the pharmacy, and provides repeated revenue stream.
Employer/ Payer	Quarterly budgeting and annual reporting encourages stricter expense management in healthcare budgets.	A healthy workforce maximizes productivity and reduces costs of healthcare long-term.	Future costs will expand as workforce ages if health is not a strategic priority for effective business operations.

Annual enrollment typically sees 20%-30% of members switch plans. [Sources: GAO analysis of Medicare enrollment data for April 2007 and the Health Resources and Services Administration's Area Resource File.]

An AstraZeneca-funded trial called SATURN that pitted AstraZeneca's cholesterol-lowering drug, Crestor, against Pfizer's cholesterol-lowering drug, Lipitor, found that Crestor failed to achieve the high levels of efficacy it had demonstrated in pivotal clinical trials.

across stakeholders of improving health outcomes rather than short-term margins. In many instances, the long-term strategy is in direct conflict with the short-term strategy, but ultimately, the long-term strategy provides incremental financial and social value through sustainable provision of quality care across the healthcare system.

This table is obviously not exhaustive. It portrays how multiple stakeholders can rally around a single business objective of healthier patients and *still* be profitable and successful. In today's market, stakeholders operate as independent units, rather than as an integrated patient-centric whole. We each have our own unique, internally focused strategies, which are usually short-term in nature and often in direct conflict with those of other organizations. **Many options exist for mutually beneficial systems, the most obvious being the shared goal of improved health outcomes for the patient**.

DELIVERING ON OUR PROMISE—WHAT MAKES PEOPLE HEALTHY?

It's worth repeating a quote from chapter 1 by the editor of the *Journal of Clinical Oncology*. Dr. Kahn from UCLA stated: "*The empirical data presented…demonstrate that brilliant laboratory and clinical breakthroughs are only the beginning of the journey toward improved population health. To complete the translation…we need to understand the types of structure and processes of care that best support the initiation of evidence-based interventions.*"[69] Dr. Kahn suggested that the role of the patient *"may be the most mutable predictor of patient outcomes."*[70] What she is saying is that we are likely to have more impact on population health by bringing scientific research to the core of patient support programs than we are by developing more advanced medicines and technologies. That's a bold statement. Despite the technological and medical advances over the past two decades, health outcomes have actually declined and the cost of care has increased. These advancements are being bottlenecked in their flow to the end user, limiting our ability to impact patients' health to the degree sought. Dr Kahn is right—we cannot progress population health without getting to a level of understanding of the patient that *explains* the structure and processes of patient thinking.

There is a growing skepticism in the healthcare industry that patient engagement is a worthwhile investment. This is an apathetic response to a plethora of badly managed efforts. The problem is not stubborn patients who cannot be moved, but our inadequate handling of them. The normative model of patient engagement today is considerably outdated. Throughout this book, several shortfalls of current approaches to healthcare have been highlighted. Interventions are not scientifically designed to create sustainable behavior change, and patients are not diagnosed to ascertain what is needed to effect cognitive change in them. A major shift in how we deliver care is undoubtedly required. The purpose of this book is to bring to light solutions for meaningful behavior change that can cause impact at a population level in a cost-effective way. This can be done under a rubric of scientific thinking with aligned evidence-based strategies and it has the potential to radically alter the delivery and outcomes of healthcare. We have only begun to scratch the surface of the patient's role in healthcare and we have yet to begin in earnest leveraging the defining fields of cognitive psychology and neuroscience to advance our understanding of patient thinking.

If we can deliver solutions that bring about meaningful behavior change effectively, the value certainly is returned. For example, in diabetes, just a 10% improvement in patients' appropriate use of recommended treatment has been shown to significantly reduce complications and cut the average annual cost of Medicare patients by 14%.[71] That creates a savings of over $3 billion annually, which, compounded over the lifetime of the patients and the growth in Medicare population, amounts to over $40 billion in 10 years.[72] That's a significant return on a relatively small improvement in patient engagement. We have not been able to deliver this impact in the costs of diabetes management nationally for the reasons already discussed in this book. However, with the right patients in the right interventions, supported by a scientifically valid and reliable platform and secure replication, such a significant impact at a national level would indeed emerge. Fortunately, the fundamentals of a strong system exist —well-educated physicians, localized convenience, accurate diagnostics and efficacious treatments.

The call to action to a more systematized and scientific approach to population management could not be more urgent. With the Medicare population on the cusp of its peak, and the incidence of disease and such risks of diseases as body mass index, or BMI, on the increase, a serious and concerted effort must be afforded to drive significant change. Every stakeholder across the complex system of healthcare has an obligation to protect the health of the population. Whether they reside in the ivory towers of the C-Suite, in the bench in R&D, at the end of a stethoscope, or in the marketing team cubicles, all constituents must take ownership of the end result —the effective progression of the health of the nation—one patient at a time.

This is not a rhetorical position. Throughout this book, the challenge has been made explicit: serious thinking, application of science, hard work, integrity to measurement, and accountability for outcomes are required in healthy doses. The industry sorely needs to sharpen its pencil and sketch out a new model of care that harnesses advances in the disciplines of cognitive science and behavior theory as the bedrock to patient and population management strategy. This book has presented a method of patient management that is rooted in science and provided a step-by-step outline for developing the approach internally. It also has presented case studies to illustrate what a new model of care can look like; provided some actionable tools to help start the process of building a business-relevant strategy around a scientific approach to population management; and shared some cautionary notes and guideposts along the way.

The administration of healthcare, the business of healthcare, and our own roles in healthcare mean nothing if we cannot deliver value on the basic premise of healthcare—*to restore or improve health*[73]. It's not rocket science, its brain science. As with any disruptive innovation, creating the ethos for change will be one of the most difficult challenges. It will necessitate leaving the status quo behind, stepping into uncomfortable newness, and holding fast to a confidence that we can deliver far beyond what we have before. It is necessary, it is our responsibility, and it is long overdue.

APPENDIX

1. WHAT IS COGNITIVE PSYCHOLOGY AND WHY IS IT IMPORTANT IN BEHAVIOR CHANGE?

The relevant fields of science to apply to patient engagement are behavioral psychology and cognitive science. The former deals with observed behavior and how the circumstances surrounding it create the behavior. The latter deals with the internal cognition, or thought processes, that direct the behavior. Cognitive science is a relatively new science, having begun in the 1960s. Its growth was a direct consequence of the "black box" in behavioral psychology. That is, the predominant premise of behavioral psychology is *describing* patterns of behavior without *explaining* the underlying mental processes that are directing the observable behavior. This is a valuable field of study, but given its limitations in being unable to explain the causes of behavior, it cannot be extended effectively into behavior change when more complex cognitive processes are driving the behavior. For example, two different people can behave similarly in the same situation but for very different reasons. An effective strategy to change the behavior of one might be

165

meaningless as a strategy to change the behavior in the other. Understanding the reasoning and how it generates the behavior is the focus of cognitive science. This field is closely linked with the field of neuroscience, in which the anatomical structures that control cognition are examined under "normal" and "non-normal" conditions. Strategy for behavior change and population management that does not do due diligence to cognitive science is unlikely to drive to measureable results.

Creating behavior change is contingent on effectively moderating the causal factors of behavior. Consequently, an organization trying to change behavior in a patient population needs to obtain a scientific model of the behavior it's trying to change. The model shouldn't focus on demographic and claims-based data (e.g., age, zip codes, the number of medications patients are taking), as those can't be modified. The scientific model should be used to validate existing patient interfacing materials and develop new elements of intervention to fill any communication gaps that might exist. The risk of proceeding without a scientifically based strategy is that the organization's efforts to change behavior likely will prove ineffective, thus providing a weak ROI and having negligible impact on population management goals.

2. WHAT EXACTLY IS A "BEHAVIORAL" PROGRAM?

Conventional programs operate at the routine level of behavior, not at the cognitive level, where the behavior is actually created, directed and changed. This is true of most programs that exist today—including many that are described as "behavioral" programs. The healthcare industry has become accepting of the premise that any program described as a "behavioral" program must be able to change behavior. The term "behavioral" is erroneously used to describe all programs that are designed to change behavior and has created a false sense of security that these programs work, when in fact most don't. To clarify, consider ADHD. A child who shows hyperactive behavior, poor concentration on homework and disruptive behavior with siblings is treated with prescription medication for his/her ADHD and a significant improvement in behavior is observed. Would you say the child's success was the result of a behavioral intervention? Of course not! The child's success was due to a pharmacological intervention. The fact that his behavior changed does not make the intervention "behavioral." A behavioral intervention is one that operates via pre-established psychological mechanisms that are at the root cause of the behavior. Such an intervention could include techniques for staying on track that operate by placing external triggers in the child's environment to replace the internal markers that are not operating effectively. In this case, both interventions would impact his behavior—but only one would be behavioral; the other would be pharmacological. In other words, a program is not "behavioral" because it impacts behavior—it is behavioral because its design is based on the root cause of the behavior. This is important is because "behavioral" programs are being sold at premium price within the healthcare industry just for carrying that label. They are justified as being "behavioral" because they are attempting to moderate "behavior," even though they haven't identified the root cause of the behavior they're trying to modify. As shown in the ADHD example, a pharmacological intervention would not be considered a behavioral intervention even though it impacts behavior. ADHD has a clear biochemical pathway behind it and prescription medication works by tapping into that mechanism of action. A behavioral intervention, similarly, works by tapping into the behavioral mechanism behind a disorder. The caution is, do not assume something called a "behavioral" intervention will change behavior. The term has been so overused it has become untrustworthy as a marker for success in behavior change. Rather, the defining factor of a real behavioral intervention is that the program has identified the root causes of the behaviors it seeks to change and has been designed to operate off those causes.

3. ARE THE REASONS FOR POOR ENGAGEMENT THE SAME ACROSS DIFFERENT CONDITIONS?

Chapter 3 described how a scientific foundation to engagement or population management strategy could be established. Table 3 in chapter 5 presented a Science Selection Tool (SST) that can be used as a starting point to help frame a scientific approach to managing different disease states. Not all diseases can be explained by the same scientific model, and patients are not equally engaged across their various conditions. For example, while the Health Belief Model has excellent application to some diseases, such as smoking cessation, other approaches have deeper and more specific application that work better with other diseases.

Importantly, every factor in these models is one that can be moderated through intervention. These models typically exclude factors such as zip code, ethnicity or socio-economic-status, since these are factors that the healthcare system cannot change. Their contribution is negligible from an applied behavior change perspective. It is interesting to note that the factors in these models vary widely from one disease to another. Patients can thus be highly engaged in one disease, but disengaged in another. These models do not suppose that a single individual must have the same engagement levels across very different disease. And even if they do have, say, 50% engagement across every disease, the reason is not necessarily the same for each disease. For example, in the case of a child with ADHD, the ability of one of the patient's caregivers (e.g., Mom) to influence the other caregiver (e.g., Dad) is a leading causal factor in determining how long the child will take ADHD medication. Compare that to oncology. The duration of therapy for a woman with breast cancer is independent of her ability to influence her spouse on treatment options. This same patient could therefore be highly engaged with her treatment for breast cancer, but woefully short on her management of her child with ADHD (due to her or her spouse's resistance). Importantly, understanding her struggle to stay engaged in treatment for her child's ADHD opens up the path to the solution: a creative piece of clear messaging designed specifically for fathers who are reluctant to treat, and have not had a firsthand conversation with the physician on the value of pharmacological management of ADHD.

Such explanatory models can also differentiate the patients across the engagement spectrum. With a full understanding of the mechanism of decision-making behind engagement, the maximum ROI is secured when the poor behavior is targeted and moderated to achieve engaged behavior. Patients targeted for intervention should be selected based on their need, which is defined as their risk for disengagement and poor outcomes. That is, the focus needs to be on shifting the bottom 20% who are creating 80% of the cost. To have a radical impact on disease outcomes and costs of care at individual *and* population levels, a dedicated strategy to modify the most costly segments cannot be ignored. Currently, we are doomed to failure as we cycle the healthier patients through costly programs and leave the patients responsible for the bulk of the problem unaddressed.

NOTES

CHAPTER 1

[1] CMS. *National Health Expenditures 2014 Highlights.* Downloaded from CMS.Gov. https://www.cms.gov/research-statistics-data-and-systems/statistics-trends-and-reports/nationalhealthexpenddata/nationalhealthaccountshistoric al.html

[2] Ibid.

[3] CMS. *National Healthcare Expenditure Data 2013.* Downloaded from CMS.Gov.

[4] CMS. *National Health Expenditures 2014 Highlights.*

[5] UNESCO Institute for Statistics. Expenditure on education as % of GDP. Online at http://data.uis.unesco.org. Accessed March, 2016.

[6] Ibid.

[7] Petersen, J. and Vuh, H. (2014). *United States: Infrastructure Investments by State Governments – Grading the Deision Process.* World Bank.

[8] World Health Organization (2003). *Adherence to Long-Term Therapies: Evidence for Action.* The World Health Report

[9] Kahn, K. (2008). Moving Research to Bench to Bedside to Community: There is still more to do. *Jl Clin Onc,* 523-526.

[10] PricewaterhouseCoopers, (2008). The price of excess: Identifying waste in healthcare spending. Online at http://www.pwc.com/us/en/healthcare/publications/the-price-of-excess.html

[11] Ibid., p.5

[12] The Kaiser Family Foundation. (2013). *Global health Facts.* Published online at http://kff.org/globaldata. Accessed September 2013

[13] National Association of Chain Drug Stores, NACDS Industry Profile 2011-2012. Online at http://www.nacds.org. Accessed September 2014

[14] PhRMA. (2007). *Drug discovery and development: Understanding the R&D process.*

[15] Ibid.

[16] Tufts Center for the Study of Drug Development. (2014). *Cost to Develop and Win Marketing Approval for a New Drug Is $2.6 Billion.* Online at http://csdd.tufts.edu/news

[17] Forbes (2013). *The Cost Of Creating A New Drug Now $5 Billion, Pushing Big Pharma To Change.* Online at http://Forbes.com

[18] DiMasi, J. (2001). Risks in new drug development: approval success rates for investigational drugs. *Clinical Pharmacology and Therapeutics, 69* (5) 297-307

CHAPTER 2

[19] Forbes, *The Cost Of Creating A New Drug Now $5 Billion*

[20] Kaiser Family Foundation and Health Research & Education Trust. (2015). *2015 Employer Health Benefits Survey.* Online at http://kff.org/health-costs/report/2015-employer-health-benefits-survey

[21] Rappleye, E. (2015) Average cost per inpatient day across 50 states. ASC Communications. www.beckershospitalreview.com/finance

[22] United States Centers for Disease Control and Prevention. Diabetes Public Health Resource: 2011 National Diabetes Fact Sheet, (2011). Available from http://www.cdc.gov/diabetes/pubs/estimates11.html

[23] Priest, J., Cantrell, C. Fincham, J. et al. (2011). Quality of Care Associated with Common Chronic Diseases in a 9-State Medicaid Population Utilizing Claims Data: An Evaluation of Medication and Health Care Use and Costs. *Population Health Management* 14(1), 43-54.

[24] United States Centers for Disease Control and Prevention. Diabetes Public Health Resource: 2014. National Diabetes Statistics Report. (2014). Available from http://www.cdc.gov/diabetes/pubs/statsreport14/national-diabetes-report-web.pdf

[25] Litzelman D., Slemenda C., et al. (1993). Reduction of lower extremity clinical abnormalities in patients with non-insulin-dependent diabetes mellitus. A randomized, controlled trial. *Ann Intern Med. 119(1):* 36-41.

[26] Ferris, F. L. (1993) How effective are treatments for diabetic retinopathy? *JAMA. 269(10):*1290-1.

[27] Okhubo, Y., Kishikawa, H. et al (1995). Intensive insulin therapy prevents the progression of diabetic microvascular complications in Japanese patients with non-insulin-dependent diabetes mellitus: a randomized prospective 6-year study. *Diabetes Res Clin Pract, 28:*103-117

[28] American Diabetes Association (2015). Microvascular Complications and Foot Care. *Diabetes Care, 38(1):*S58–S66

[29] American Diabetes Association (2013). The cost of Diabetes. Available at http://www.diabetes.org/advocacy/news-events/cost-of-diabetes.html

[30] Unitedhealth Group. (2010). *The United States of Diabetes: New Report Shows Half the Country Could Have Diabetes or Prediabetes at a Cost of $3.35 Trillion by 2020.* Available at htttp://www.unitedhealthgroup.com/newsroom/articles/news/unitedhealth

[31] WHO, *Adherence to Long-Term Therapies: Evidence for Action*

[32] Kahn, *Moving Research to Bedside to Community*

[33] Partridge, A., LaFountain, A. et al. (2008). Adherence to Adherence to Initial Adjuvant Anastrozole Therapy Among Women With Early-Stage Breast Cancer. *JCO, 28(4):*556-562

[34] Ibid.

[35] Briesacher, B., Andrade, S., et al, (2008). Comparison of drug adherence rates among patients with seven different medical conditions. *Pharmacotherapy, 28(4):*437-443

[36] Lasmar L, Camargos P, Champs N, et al. (2009). Adherence rates to inhaled corticosteroids and their impact on asthma control. *Allergy, 64(5)*:784-789

[37] Briesacher, B., Andrade, S., et al, *Comparison of drug adherence rates*

[38] Ibid.

[39] Mind Field Solutions. (2016) *The Cost of Failure.* Data on file.

[40] Ibid.

[41] NEHI. (2009). *Thinking Outside the Pillbox: A System-wide Approach to Improving Patient Medication Adherence for Chronic Disease.* A NEHI Research Brief.

[42] Kahn, *Moving Research to Bedside to Community*

[43] Ariely, D. (2008). *Predictably Irrational: The hidden forces that shape our decisions.* New York, Harper Collins

[44] Kahn, *Moving Research to Bedside to Community* p.525

[45] Ibid.

[46] Burgess, P. (1997). Theory and Methodology in Executive Function Research. In: *Methodology of Frontal and Executive Function.* P. Rabbitt (Ed.). UK, Psychology Press

[47] Moran, A. (1999). *Fractionation of the Executive System: Theoretical, Statistical and Behavioural Components.* PhD Thesis, University of Liverpool, UK.

[48] Norman, D. and Shallice, T. (1980). Attention to action: willed and automatic control of behavior. Center for Human Information Processing (Technical Report No.99). Reprinted in revised form in R.J. Davidson et al (Eds.) (1986), *Consciousness and self regulation, Vol. 4.* New York, Plenum Press.

[49] Shallice, T. and Burgess, P. 1991. Higher order cognitive impairments and frontal lobe lesions in man. In H. S. Levin et al (Eds) *Frontal lobe function and dysfunction* (pp. 125-138). New York, Oxford University Press

CHAPTER 4

[50] Prochaska and Norcross, *Stages of change*

[51] CMS. *National Health Expenditures 2014 Highlights*

[52] Partridge, LaFountain, et al. *Adherence to Initial Adjuvant Anastrozole Therapy*

[53] Mind Field Solutions, *The Cost of Failure*

[54] Prochaska, J. & Norcross, J. (2002). Stages of change. In J. C. Norcross (Ed.), *Psychotherapy relationships that work* 303-310. Oxford University Press, New York

[55] Jesus Christ. Matthew 2:17, NIV Bible translation.

[56] Ibid.

[57] Hibbard, J., Stockard, J., Mahoney, E, & Tusler, M. (2004). Development of the Patient Activation Measure (PAM): Conceptualizing and Measuring Activation in Patients and Consumers. *HSR: 39(4):*1005-1026

[58] Unitedhealth Center for Health Reform and Modernization (2010). *United States of Diabetes: Challenges and opportunities in the decade ahead.* http://www.unitedhealthgroup.com/~/media/uhg/pdf/2010/unh-working-paper-5.ashx

[59] Ibid.

[60] Unitedhealth Center for Health Reform and Modernization, *United States of Diabetes*

[61] Partridge, LaFountain et al, *Adherence to Initial Adjuvant Anastrozole Therapy*

CHAPTER 9

[62] H. James Harrington. (1991). *Business Process Improvement: The Breakthrough Strategy for Total Quality, Productivity, and Competitiveness.* McGraw Hill. p.164

CHAPTER 10

---

[63] CMS. *National Health Expenditures 2014 Highlights*

[64] Kaiser Family Foundation, *2015 Employer Health Benefits Survey.*

[65] Ibid.

CHAPTER 11

---

[66] Merrian-Webster dictionary. Online at www.merrian-webster.com

[67] WHO, *Adherence to Long-Term Therapies*

[68] Dunbar-Jacob, J. & Mortimer-Stephens, M. (2001). Treatment adherence in chronic disease. *J Clin Epidemiol. 54*:S57-60

[69] Kahn, *Moving Research to Bedside to Community*

[70] Ibid., 524

[71] Mind Field Solutions, *The Cost of Failure*

[72] Ibid.

[73] Merrian-Webster dictionary